THE CORTISOL DETOX DIET PLAN

Free Your Body in 28-Days From Bad Stress and Stubborn Fat. A Proven Method to Regain Your Vitality and Feel Your Best.

JENNA SWIFT

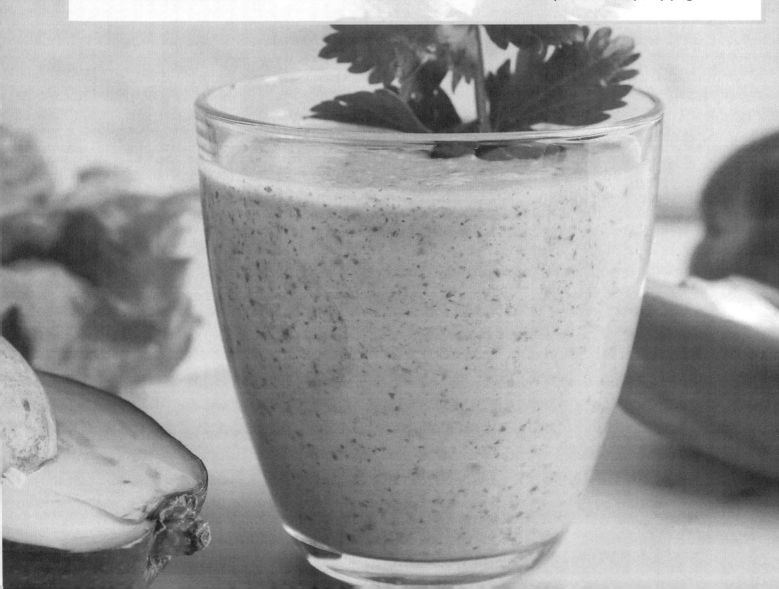

Table of Contents

CHAPTER 8
SNACK RECIPES

CHAPTER 9
NOURISHING FOODS TO BALANCE CORTISOL

CHAPTER 10
STABILIZING BLOOD SUGAR FOR WEIGHT LOSS

CHAPTER 11
HYDRATION AND CORTISOL REDUCTION

How to Break Free from Bad Stress and Restore Your Vitality

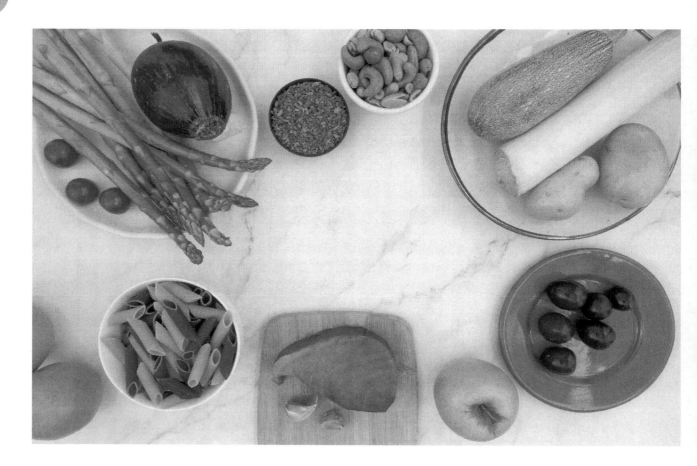

Understanding Cortisol and Its Role in Your Health

Cortisol is often referred to as the "stress hormone," but its role in your body goes far beyond just reacting to stress. It is a hormone produced by your adrenal glands, small organs located just above your kidneys, and is crucial for various functions in your body. While cortisol is necessary for survival, chronic high levels can become harmful, leading to a range of health issues. Understanding how cortisol works, its impact on your body, and why managing its levels is essential can provide you with the foundation needed to regain control of your health and well-being.

What Exactly Is Cortisol?

Cortisol is part of the body's *endocrine system* and plays a vital role in maintaining homeostasis, the body's internal balance. It is released during times of stress or low blood sugar to help your body manage the situation, allowing you to respond quickly and effectively. In short bursts, cortisol is beneficial and essential for survival, but the problem arises when cortisol is elevated for too long.

Key functions of cortisol include:

- **Regulating metabolism**: Cortisol helps control how your body uses carbohydrates, fats, and proteins for energy. When cortisol levels are balanced, your body can efficiently process nutrients to keep you energized.

- **Managing inflammation**: Cortisol helps reduce inflammation and regulates your immune response. It's part of your body's natural healing process, but chronic high cortisol can suppress your immune function, making you more susceptible to illness.

- **Controlling blood sugar levels**: During stressful situations, cortisol increases blood sugar levels to provide immediate energy. While helpful in the short term, persistently high cortisol can cause insulin resistance and lead to weight gain, especially around the belly area.

- **Supporting the sleep-wake cycle**: Cortisol levels naturally fluctuate throughout the day, typically peaking in the morning to help wake you up and declining in the evening to prepare your body for sleep.

Cortisol and the Stress Response

When you encounter stress—whether it's physical, emotional, or psychological—your body activates what's known as the **fight-or-flight response**. This is where cortisol shines: It helps you respond to immediate danger by releasing glucose into your bloodstream for quick energy, increasing your heart rate, and sharpening your focus.

Once the perceived threat is gone, cortisol levels should drop, and your body returns to its normal state. But in today's fast-paced world, stress is often constant. From work deadlines to family pressures, your body may stay in a state of heightened cortisol production, even when there's no immediate physical danger. This can lead to a *chronic stress response*, which is damaging over time.

The Long-Term Effects of Elevated Cortisol

When cortisol levels remain elevated for an extended period, your body begins to suffer. Chronic high cortisol can lead to:

- **Weight gain**, particularly around the abdominal area, which is known as "stress belly." This type of fat is not only stubborn but also more dangerous, as it increases the risk of heart disease and diabetes.

- **Sleep disturbances**, such as trouble falling asleep, waking up frequently during the night, or experiencing early-morning insomnia. High cortisol levels disrupt the normal sleep-wake cycle, leaving you feeling tired and drained during the day.

- **Mood swings and irritability**: Excessive cortisol can lead to feelings of anxiety, irritability, and even depression. It impacts neurotransmitter balance, making it harder for you to manage your emotions effectively.

- **Reduced immune function**: Over time, elevated cortisol can suppress your immune system, making you more vulnerable to infections and illnesses.

- **Blood sugar imbalances**: Since cortisol raises blood sugar levels, consistently high cortisol can increase the risk of insulin resistance and type 2 diabetes.
- **Muscle weakness and fatigue**: Cortisol breaks down protein in your muscles to provide energy during stressful times. Prolonged elevated cortisol can lead to muscle breakdown, leaving you feeling weak and fatigued.

How to Know if Your Cortisol Is Out of Balance

If you're feeling overwhelmed, exhausted, and struggling to lose weight, it's possible that cortisol could be to blame. While lab tests can confirm elevated cortisol levels, there are several signs that your cortisol may be out of balance:

- **Unexplained weight gain**, especially around the midsection
- **Constant fatigue**, even after a full night's sleep
- **Difficulty sleeping** or frequent waking during the night
- **Increased cravings** for sugary or salty foods
- **Frequent mood swings**, irritability, or anxiety
- **Reduced immunity**, such as frequent colds or infections
- **Low energy** and difficulty concentrating

If you recognize these symptoms, managing cortisol through lifestyle changes is crucial to restoring balance in your body and regaining your health.

Why Managing Cortisol Is Key to Long-Term Health

Balanced cortisol levels are essential for maintaining good health. Cortisol itself is not the enemy—it's your body's way of protecting you from immediate threats and maintaining equilibrium. But when cortisol levels remain elevated for too long, your body enters a state of chronic stress that leads to a variety of health problems.

By understanding cortisol's role and impact on your body, you can begin taking steps to manage its levels. Diet, exercise, sleep, and stress management all play a role in bringing cortisol back into balance. This book will guide you through these steps, offering practical solutions designed to help you lower cortisol, lose stubborn fat, and reclaim your energy.

The Science of Stress and Weight Gain

Stress is a natural part of life, and your body is designed to handle it in short bursts. However, when stress becomes chronic, it triggers a cascade of hormonal responses that can severely impact your health, including weight gain. Understanding the connection between stress, cortisol, and weight gain is critical to taking control of your body and breaking the cycle of stress-induced fat accumulation, particularly around the belly.

How Stress Affects Your Body

When you experience stress—whether it's a looming work deadline, family pressures, or emotional challenges—your body activates what's called the **fight-or-flight response**. This response is designed to help you deal with immediate threats by releasing hormones like **adrenaline** and **cortisol**.

Cortisol plays a central role in this process. It prepares your body to respond to the stressor by raising your blood sugar levels, increasing your energy supply, and suppressing non-essential functions like digestion and reproduction. This is beneficial when you need to act quickly to handle a short-term threat. But when stress is constant, cortisol remains elevated, and that's where the trouble begins.

- **Constant sugar spikes**: Cortisol releases glucose into your bloodstream to provide energy. But if you're not physically burning that energy—because your stress isn't coming from a physical threat—those elevated glucose levels are stored as fat.
- **Fat storage, especially in the abdomen**: Chronic high cortisol leads to fat being stored in the belly area, known as visceral fat, which is not only difficult to lose but also dangerous. It's associated with a higher risk of heart disease, type 2 diabetes, and other health conditions.

The Role of Cortisol in Weight Gain

One of cortisol's primary functions is to increase your body's energy supply in response to stress. It does this by converting stored glycogen into glucose, which can be quickly used for energy. But if this energy isn't used—like in the case of mental stress from work or life challenges—it leads to:

- **Increased fat storage**: Your body stores unused glucose as fat, primarily around the abdomen. This fat is more metabolically active, meaning it produces more stress hormones and perpetuates a cycle of stress and fat accumulation.
- **Increased cravings**: High cortisol levels make you crave high-calorie, sugary, and salty foods, which provide quick energy. This leads to overeating and can further contribute to weight gain.

Insulin Resistance and Weight Gain

Another significant effect of chronic stress and elevated cortisol is its impact on **insulin**—the hormone responsible for regulating blood sugar levels. When your cortisol levels are constantly high, your cells become less sensitive to insulin, leading to **insulin resistance**. This means that glucose is less efficiently absorbed by your cells and stays in your bloodstream longer, prompting your body to produce more insulin.

Here's what happens next:

- **More fat storage**: Elevated insulin causes your body to store more fat, particularly in the abdominal area.
- **Difficulty losing weight**: Insulin resistance makes it harder for your body to burn fat, even when you're eating less or exercising.
- **Energy crashes**: As blood sugar fluctuates due to insulin resistance, you experience energy crashes that leave you feeling fatigued and craving more sugar, creating a vicious cycle of weight gain and stress.

Stress, Sleep, and Weight Gain

High cortisol levels don't just affect your metabolism—they also interfere with your sleep patterns, leading to further weight gain. Cortisol follows a natural rhythm, rising in the morning to wake you up and gradually declining throughout the day to help you wind down and sleep. But when stress is constant, cortisol levels stay elevated at night, disrupting your ability to fall asleep and stay asleep.

Here's how poor sleep ties into weight gain:

- **Increased hunger hormones**: Lack of sleep increases the production of **ghrelin**, the hormone that makes you feel hungry, and decreases **leptin**, the hormone that signals fullness. This imbalance leads to overeating and poor food choices.
- **Slower metabolism**: Inadequate sleep slows down your metabolism, making it harder to burn calories. Combined with increased appetite, this creates the perfect storm for weight gain.
- **Impaired decision-making**: Sleep deprivation impairs your judgment and self-control, making it more likely that you'll reach for sugary or processed foods instead of healthier options.

The Vicious Cycle of Stress and Weight Gain

Chronic stress creates a **vicious cycle** that's difficult to break. High cortisol levels lead to overeating, especially foods high in sugar and fat, which in turn lead to weight gain. This weight gain, particularly around the belly, increases cortisol production, perpetuating the cycle.

- **Emotional eating**: Stress often triggers emotional eating, where food is used as a coping mechanism for dealing with stress. This results in excessive calorie intake and further weight gain.
- **Body image and self-esteem**: As weight increases, many people experience lower self-esteem and body image issues, which can lead to more stress, compounding the problem.

This cycle is not just a result of poor willpower or lack of discipline. It's a biological response to chronic stress, and it's one of the reasons why many women struggle to lose weight despite their best efforts.

Breaking the Cycle

Breaking this cycle starts with understanding how stress affects your body and making lifestyle changes to manage it. Learning to balance cortisol levels through diet, exercise, and proper sleep can help you regain control over your weight and overall health. You'll find that once cortisol levels start to normalize, your cravings decrease, your energy stabilizes, and your body becomes more responsive to healthy changes, allowing you to finally break free from stress-induced weight gain.

How Chronic Stress Impacts Your Vitality

Stress is not just something that affects you emotionally; it has profound physical consequences that drain your energy, leaving you feeling constantly fatigued and disconnected from your sense of vitality. When stress becomes chronic, the effects can slowly chip away at your well-being. This kind of ongoing, relentless stress can lead to a range of physical, emotional, and mental problems that may feel like they're out of your control. However, by understanding how chronic stress impacts your body and mind, you can begin to take back control and regain the energy you need to thrive.

The Energy Drain: How Stress Saps Your Vitality

When you're constantly stressed, your body is always in a state of **high alert**. This means your fight-or-flight response is continually activated, keeping your cortisol levels elevated. Cortisol is useful in small doses—it helps you respond to immediate danger by giving you a quick burst of energy. But when your body is producing too much cortisol, day in and day out, it starts to have the opposite effect, draining your energy reserves.

Here's how chronic stress depletes your energy:

- **Constant cortisol production:** Your adrenal glands, which produce cortisol, get overworked. The body can't sustain this level of output without consequences. Over time, your adrenal function becomes compromised, leaving you feeling constantly tired, no matter how much sleep you get.
- **Nutrient depletion:** Chronic stress forces your body to use more vitamins and minerals, especially B vitamins, magnesium, and vitamin C. These nutrients are crucial for energy production and mood regulation. When they're depleted, it becomes harder to feel energized and balanced.
- **Disrupted sleep patterns:** Elevated cortisol levels interfere with your ability to fall asleep and stay asleep. Sleep is your body's way of recovering and replenishing energy. Without proper rest, you start every day at a deficit, feeling drained from the moment you wake up.

The Emotional Impact of Chronic Stress

Beyond physical exhaustion, chronic stress also takes a toll on your **emotional well-being**. Constant high levels of stress can lead to anxiety, irritability, and even depression. When your body is under prolonged stress, it disrupts the balance of important neurotransmitters like serotonin and dopamine, which are responsible for regulating your mood.

- **Anxiety and worry:** With cortisol levels elevated, your mind can become stuck in a state of hyper-vigilance, making it difficult to relax or focus. You may find yourself constantly worrying, feeling anxious about both small and large issues.
- **Mood swings:** You might notice that you're more irritable or easily frustrated. This isn't just in your head—chronic stress physically alters your brain's ability to regulate emotions. Small inconveniences may start to feel overwhelming, and you might find yourself snapping at others or feeling out of control emotionally.
- **Feelings of hopelessness:** Prolonged exposure to stress can also lead to feelings of helplessness or burnout. This emotional exhaustion makes it difficult to see a way out of your situation, compounding the physical exhaustion that stress already causes.

How Chronic Stress Impacts Your Physical Health

When stress becomes chronic, it doesn't just affect your energy levels and emotional state—it can also manifest as **physical health problems**. This is because cortisol, while necessary in small amounts, has destructive effects when it remains elevated for too long.

- **Immune system suppression:** High cortisol levels suppress the immune system, making it harder for your body to fight off infections. You might find that you catch colds more often or take longer to recover from illnesses.
- **Inflammation:** Chronic stress leads to increased inflammation in the body, which is a contributing factor to numerous health issues, including heart disease, arthritis, and digestive disorders.
- **Increased blood pressure and heart rate:** Stress causes your heart to work harder, and over time, this can lead to **hypertension** (high blood pressure), increasing your risk of cardiovascular diseases.
- **Digestive issues:** Cortisol diverts energy away from non-essential systems, including digestion. As a result, chronic stress can lead to problems like indigestion, bloating, constipation, or even irritable bowel syndrome (IBS).

The Vicious Cycle of Stress and Fatigue

One of the most frustrating aspects of chronic stress is the **cycle of fatigue** it creates. When you're stressed, your body uses more energy and resources just to keep up. But the more energy you expend, the more fatigued you become, leading to a situation where you feel too tired to make the lifestyle changes needed to reduce stress. It's a cycle that can feel impossible to break:

- **Stress leads to exhaustion**: Elevated cortisol disrupts sleep and drains your energy, making you feel constantly tired.

- **Exhaustion makes it harder to manage stress**: When you're tired, your ability to cope with stress diminishes, making even small stressors feel overwhelming.

- **Stress becomes harder to manage**: Without the energy to deal with stress effectively, it builds up, leading to even more fatigue and further depleting your vitality.

Stress and Weight Gain: Another Layer to the Fatigue

To make matters worse, chronic stress often leads to **weight gain**, particularly in the abdominal area. This is because cortisol increases fat storage, particularly visceral fat, which surrounds your internal organs and is harder to lose. The additional weight puts more strain on your body, exacerbating feelings of fatigue and making physical activity more challenging.

Moreover, when you're tired and stressed, you're more likely to reach for **unhealthy foods** like sugar and processed snacks to give you a temporary energy boost. But these quick fixes only contribute to more weight gain, blood sugar imbalances, and the cycle of fatigue.

By understanding how chronic stress impacts every aspect of your vitality, you can start to take the steps necessary to break free from the cycle of exhaustion and reclaim your energy.

Who This Book Is For: A Practical, Proven Solution for Busy Women

This book is designed for women who are juggling the relentless demands of work, family, and personal commitments, and yet find themselves drained of energy and struggling with stubborn weight gain. It's for those who feel like they've tried every diet and workout plan, only to be met with frustration. It's for the woman who wakes up tired, fights through her day with caffeine and sugar, and wonders why, despite her best efforts, she can't seem to lose the weight that seems to cling to her midsection.

If you see yourself in any of these descriptions, this book is written for you.

The Busy Professional Woman

Are you constantly on the go, running from one meeting to the next, trying to balance deadlines with your personal life? If you're a professional woman who feels like there's never enough time in the day, you're probably no stranger to stress. It creeps into every aspect of your life, from that project at work you can't stop thinking about to the endless emails you feel obligated to check, even late at night.

You might have noticed that all this stress has taken a toll on your body. You're exhausted, even after a full night's sleep, and you've gained weight, especially around your belly, despite your best attempts to eat well and stay active. This book offers you practical, time-saving solutions that fit into your hectic lifestyle—simple changes that make a big impact on your cortisol levels, your energy, and your waistline.

- **Quick meal prep tips**: Recipes and meal plans designed to save you time while supporting cortisol balance.
- **Efficient stress-reducing techniques**: Methods that help lower your stress without adding more tasks to your already full plate.
- **Short, effective workouts**: Exercise plans that don't require hours at the gym but still help you lose weight and feel energized.

The Stressed-Out Mom

You love your family, but the constant demands of motherhood have left you feeling burnt out. Between taking care of the kids, managing the household, and trying to keep up with your own needs, it feels like there's no room to breathe. You're always "on," always in caregiver mode, and always putting yourself last. The result? You feel drained and overwhelmed. You've noticed that you've gained weight, particularly around your belly, and no matter what you try, you can't seem to get rid of it.

If you're a mom who feels like her stress levels are off the charts and you're desperate for a solution that doesn't require hours of your time, this book is for you. We understand that you're busy and that your days are unpredictable. That's why this program is designed to be flexible and forgiving, offering small but powerful changes you can make in your life that will help you feel better, sleep better, and regain control over your health.

- **Family-friendly recipes**: Meals that your whole family will enjoy, helping you stay on track without having to cook separate meals.
- **Simple routines**: Stress-management techniques you can do in just a few minutes a day.
- **Actionable tips**: Easy-to-implement strategies for reducing stress and increasing energy, even on the busiest of days.

The Woman Struggling with Weight Loss

Are you frustrated because no matter how much you diet or exercise, the weight just won't come off? Perhaps you've noticed that despite your efforts, the fat around your belly seems to get worse when you're stressed. That's because high cortisol levels, which are triggered by stress, signal your body to store fat, especially in the abdominal area.

This book offers a solution that goes beyond the usual "eat less, move more" advice. It's not about starving yourself or doing hours of cardio. Instead, it's about understanding the role that cortisol plays in your weight loss struggles and learning how to bring it back into balance. Once you do, your body will respond more positively to healthy eating and exercise, and you'll finally start to see the results you've been working so hard for.

- **Cortisol-balancing foods**: Learn which foods naturally lower cortisol and promote weight loss.
- **Stress-free exercise**: Discover low-impact workouts that help you burn fat without increasing stress levels.
- **Long-term results**: Strategies that help you keep the weight off by managing stress in sustainable, realistic ways.

The Woman Ready for a Sustainable Change

This book is also for the woman who's tired of quick fixes and fad diets that leave her feeling deprived and exhausted. If you're looking for a **practical, proven solution** that addresses the root cause of your weight gain and lack of energy, you've come to the right place. The **Cortisol Detox Diet Plan** is not just another weight loss program. It's a comprehensive approach to healing your body from the inside out, helping you feel energized, focused, and in control of your life again.

Whether you're a busy professional, a mom, or someone simply seeking a sustainable solution to stress and weight management, this book provides you with the tools you need to succeed. The steps are simple, but the impact will be profound, helping you regain your vitality, manage your stress, and finally lose that stubborn weight.

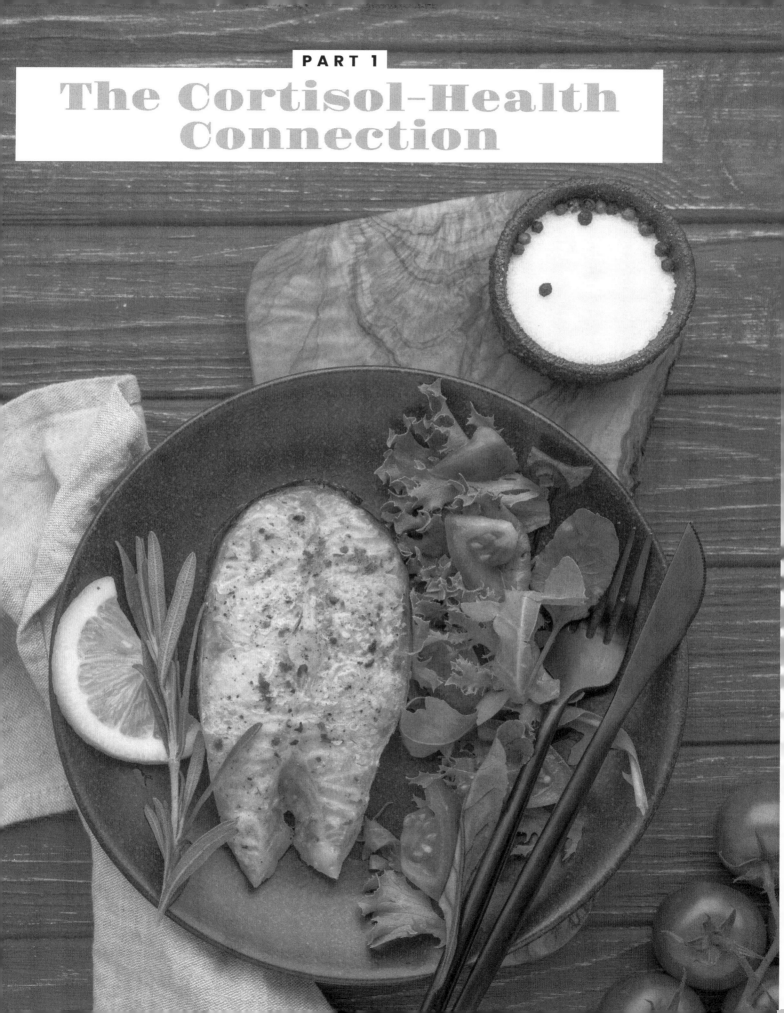

PART 1

The Cortisol-Health Connection

CHAPTER 1

What Is Cortisol?

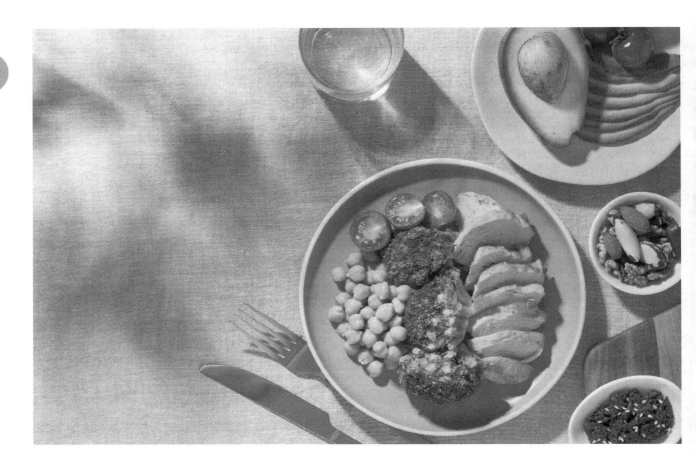

Why Cortisol Is Known as the "Stress Hormone"

Cortisol has earned the nickname "the stress hormone" for a very good reason. It is the primary hormone your body produces in response to stress, and it plays a vital role in helping you handle stressful situations. Released by the adrenal glands, cortisol is part of the body's **fight-or-flight** response, a survival mechanism that's been with us since ancient times. In a moment of crisis, cortisol surges through your system, giving you the energy and focus you need to overcome challenges or escape danger. However, when stress becomes chronic, the same cortisol that once helped you can turn into a harmful force that damages your health and well-being.

The Role of Cortisol in the Fight-or-Flight Response

When you encounter a stressful situation—whether it's physical, emotional, or psychological—your body activates its **sympathetic nervous system** to prepare you for action. This system triggers the release of cortisol along with other hormones like adrenaline. Cortisol's primary role is to make sure you have enough energy to respond to the threat.

- **Increased glucose levels**: Cortisol prompts your liver to release glucose into your bloodstream, providing a rapid energy source for your muscles and brain. This ensures that you can fight off the danger or flee if necessary.
- **Suppression of non-essential functions**: To conserve energy for immediate use, cortisol temporarily shuts down bodily systems that aren't critical in a life-or-death situation, such as digestion, reproduction, and immune function.
- **Enhanced focus and alertness**: Cortisol increases your focus and sharpens your senses, helping you react more effectively to whatever is causing the stress.

This fight-or-flight response was essential in ancient times when humans frequently faced physical threats. But in modern life, the stresses we encounter are more likely to be mental or emotional—work deadlines, financial concerns, family pressures—yet the body reacts in the same way as if it were preparing for physical danger.

The Problem with Chronic Stress

In a short-term, immediate crisis, cortisol is helpful. Once the threat is gone, cortisol levels naturally decrease, allowing your body to return to normal. However, when stress becomes **chronic**, cortisol levels remain elevated for extended periods, which is when problems begin to arise.

Constantly high cortisol levels can:

- **Disrupt your sleep**: Cortisol is supposed to follow a natural rhythm, peaking in the morning to wake you up and gradually declining throughout the day. But if you're under constant stress, cortisol levels stay high at night, leading to trouble falling asleep or waking up in the middle of the night.
- **Weaken your immune system**: Prolonged high cortisol suppresses immune function, making you more susceptible to colds, infections, and even more serious illnesses.
- **Cause weight gain**: Cortisol increases fat storage, particularly in the abdominal area, where fat cells have more cortisol receptors. This "stress belly" is not only frustrating but also more dangerous, as it's linked to a higher risk of heart disease and diabetes.

Why Does Your Body Produce So Much Cortisol Under Stress?

Your body produces cortisol as a survival mechanism, ensuring that you have the energy to tackle whatever is threatening your well-being. When faced with a perceived threat, cortisol ensures you're equipped with the resources to respond effectively. But your body doesn't distinguish between a physical threat—like being chased by a wild animal—and a modern stressor—like a looming work deadline. Both trigger the same hormonal response.

- **Modern life equals constant stress**: The pressures of modern living—multitasking, balancing work and home life, managing financial obligations—mean that your body often operates in a constant state of low-level stress. Your cortisol never has the chance to return to baseline, leading to a cycle of chronic stress and consistently elevated cortisol levels.
- **Cortisol and mental stress**: Interestingly, the body reacts similarly to emotional stress. If you're worrying about an argument with a loved one, experiencing anxiety, or feeling overwhelmed by work responsibilities, your cortisol levels spike in the same way they would if you were facing physical danger.

The Double-Edged Sword of Cortisol

While cortisol is essential for survival, it can also be a **double-edged sword**. When used appropriately, cortisol gives you the burst of energy and focus needed to handle challenges. But when cortisol is overproduced due to prolonged stress, it begins to have negative effects on the body, causing a range of health issues.

- **Mood and mental health**: High cortisol levels are linked to anxiety, depression, and irritability. This happens because cortisol interferes with neurotransmitters in the brain, including serotonin, which helps regulate mood.
- **Energy crashes**: After the initial surge of energy cortisol provides, you may experience significant crashes. These energy dips can leave you feeling drained and may lead to increased cravings for sugar and caffeine, further perpetuating the cycle of stress.
- **Impact on the heart**: Chronic high cortisol levels can increase blood pressure, strain the heart, and lead to long-term cardiovascular issues. Stress hormones like cortisol prompt the heart to work harder, which, over time, can damage your heart health.

The Balance Between Cortisol and Relaxation

It's important to note that cortisol itself isn't inherently bad. In fact, you need cortisol to function properly. It's essential for waking you up in the morning, managing your energy levels throughout the day, and keeping you alert and focused. The key is finding balance.

- **Stress management**: This book will guide you through effective stress management techniques that help lower cortisol to healthy levels, ensuring that you're not living in a constant state of fight-or-flight.
- **Creating a rhythm**: By supporting your body's natural cortisol rhythm through diet, sleep, and stress-reduction strategies, you can regain balance and energy, avoiding the damaging effects of chronically elevated cortisol.

Understanding why cortisol is called the "stress hormone" is the first step in recognizing how it impacts your health. By learning to manage stress, you can bring your cortisol levels back into balance, allowing you to live with more energy, better health, and less stress.

How Elevated Cortisol Affects Your Weight and Health

Elevated cortisol is often the missing link in weight loss struggles and overall health issues, especially when stress becomes a constant part of life. Cortisol is a hormone produced by the adrenal glands, and it plays a key role in various bodily functions, including metabolism, immune response, and the regulation of blood sugar. When you're under stress, your body produces cortisol to help you cope. While this response is beneficial in the short term, chronic stress leads to prolonged elevated cortisol levels, which can negatively affect your weight and health in multiple ways.

Cortisol and Fat Storage

When cortisol levels remain high for an extended period, your body enters a state where it favors **fat storage**, especially in the abdominal area. This phenomenon occurs because cortisol triggers the release of glucose (sugar) into the bloodstream to provide energy for the fight-or-flight response. However, when you don't use this energy (which is often the case in modern stress situations where the threat is emotional or psychological rather than physical), your body stores the excess glucose as fat.

- **Belly fat and cortisol**: Cortisol has a specific impact on visceral fat—the type of fat that surrounds your internal organs. This "stress belly" is particularly harmful because it increases the risk of developing serious health conditions, such as heart disease, diabetes, and metabolic syndrome. Unfortunately, this kind of fat is also the most stubborn to lose.

- **Insulin resistance**: Elevated cortisol can lead to insulin resistance. When your cells become less responsive to insulin, your body compensates by producing more of it, causing glucose to stay in your bloodstream longer. This leads to more fat storage and makes weight loss even more difficult.

The Impact on Metabolism

One of cortisol's primary roles is to regulate how your body uses energy. When cortisol levels are balanced, your metabolism functions efficiently, converting food into energy and keeping you active throughout the day. However, when cortisol remains elevated for long periods, it disrupts your metabolism, making it harder to lose weight and easier to gain it.

Here's how elevated cortisol slows your metabolism:

- **Muscle breakdown**: Cortisol breaks down muscle tissue to produce glucose. While this may provide short-term energy during stressful situations, over time, it leads to a loss of lean muscle mass. Since muscle is metabolically active, the less muscle you have, the fewer calories you burn at rest.

- **Fat storage mode**: Your body perceives chronic stress as a threat, and elevated cortisol signals your system to store fat as a protective measure. This shift in metabolism ensures that your body has enough resources to handle the perceived threat, but in today's world, this often results in weight gain rather than survival.

Cravings and Overeating

If you've ever found yourself reaching for comfort foods during stressful times, you're not alone. Elevated cortisol has a direct impact on your appetite and cravings, driving you to consume more calories, particularly from foods high in sugar and fat.

- **Increased hunger**: Cortisol stimulates your appetite as part of its role in preparing your body for a fight-or-flight response. After all, if you were running from danger, you'd need a quick energy source. Unfortunately, in the context of everyday stress, this leads to unnecessary calorie consumption, especially when combined with the convenience of high-calorie, processed foods.

- **Emotional eating**: Elevated cortisol not only increases physical hunger but also triggers emotional eating. Stress can cause you to seek comfort in food, especially sugary and fatty foods, which temporarily boost levels of serotonin—a neurotransmitter that helps regulate mood. This can create a cycle of stress eating that leads to further weight gain.

How Cortisol Affects Sleep and Weight

Sleep is one of the most important factors for maintaining a healthy weight, but elevated cortisol interferes with your sleep patterns. Normally, cortisol follows a **diurnal rhythm**, meaning it peaks in the morning to wake you up and gradually decreases throughout the day, reaching its lowest point at night. However, when you're chronically stressed, cortisol levels may remain elevated in the evening, disrupting your ability to fall asleep and stay asleep.

- **Sleep deprivation and weight gain**: Lack of sleep leads to increased production of ghrelin (the hormone that stimulates hunger) and decreased production of leptin (the hormone that signals fullness). This imbalance causes you to feel hungrier during the day and more likely to overeat.
- **Cortisol and nighttime wakefulness**: Elevated cortisol levels at night can cause you to wake up frequently or too early in the morning, preventing you from getting restorative sleep. Poor sleep leads to fatigue and low energy during the day, making it harder to stay active and burn calories.

Long-Term Health Consequences

The effects of chronically elevated cortisol extend far beyond weight gain. Over time, high cortisol levels can lead to a host of health problems that affect both your physical and mental well-being.

- **Weakened immune system**: Cortisol suppresses immune function, making you more susceptible to illnesses like colds, infections, and even more serious conditions over time.
- **Cardiovascular issues**: Prolonged elevated cortisol increases your risk of high blood pressure and heart disease. Stress hormones prompt your heart to work harder, which can eventually lead to long-term damage.
- **Mental health struggles**: High cortisol levels are linked to anxiety, depression, and mood swings. Cortisol disrupts the balance of neurotransmitters in the brain, making it harder to manage stress and regulate emotions.

Breaking the Cycle

Breaking free from the effects of elevated cortisol on your weight and health requires a multi-faceted approach. Diet, exercise, sleep, and stress management all play crucial roles in reducing cortisol levels and helping your body return to a state of balance. By addressing these areas, you can begin to reverse the negative impact of chronic stress on your weight and health, regaining control over your body and your life.

CHAPTER 2

The Link Between Cortisol and Stubborn Fat

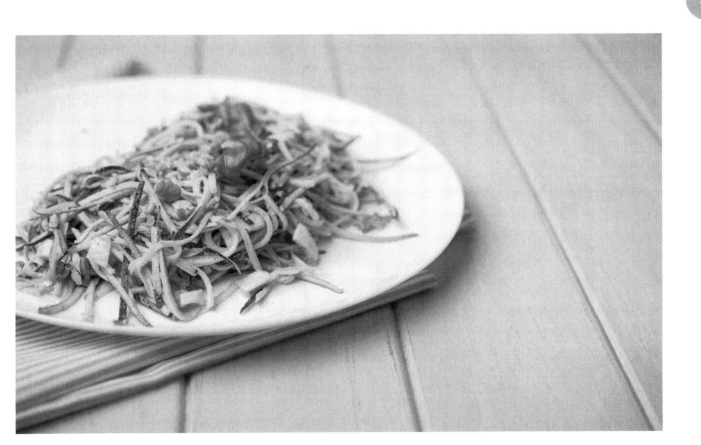

Why Belly Fat Is Linked to High Cortisol Levels

If you've been struggling with stubborn belly fat despite making changes to your diet and exercise routine, cortisol may be the missing piece of the puzzle. Often called the "stress hormone," cortisol is produced by your adrenal glands in response to stress. While it's essential for handling short-term stressors, chronic elevated cortisol can have lasting effects on your body, especially when it comes to fat storage in the abdominal area.

The Cortisol-Belly Fat Connection

When you're under stress, your body releases cortisol to help you manage the situation. This hormonal response evolved as a survival mechanism, giving you the energy to react to physical threats. However, in modern life, stress is often emotional or psychological—caused by work pressures, financial worries, or family responsibilities. Your body doesn't distinguish between these forms of stress and physical danger, so it produces cortisol in both situations.

Cortisol's main job is to ensure you have enough energy to cope with the stressor. It does this by:

- **Releasing glucose into your bloodstream**: Cortisol increases your blood sugar levels to provide quick energy. If you were fleeing from a threat, this would help fuel your muscles. But when stress is mental or emotional, and you're not using that glucose for physical activity, your body stores the excess as fat.

- **Promoting fat storage**: Cortisol encourages the storage of fat, particularly in the abdominal area. Belly fat, also known as visceral fat, surrounds vital organs and is more metabolically active than fat in other parts of the body. This means it can release more inflammatory markers and stress hormones, perpetuating the cycle of stress and fat accumulation.

Why Belly Fat Is Particularly Sensitive to Cortisol

Your abdominal area has a high concentration of **cortisol receptors**, making it especially sensitive to the effects of this hormone. When cortisol levels are elevated for extended periods, your body prioritizes fat storage in the belly as a way to protect itself. The fat around your organs can serve as a quick energy reserve, which would have been helpful in prehistoric times when food was scarce and survival was uncertain.

In today's world, however, this mechanism works against you. Even if you're eating relatively well and exercising, high cortisol levels can keep your body in fat-storage mode, particularly around your waistline. This explains why you might notice fat accumulating in your midsection despite your best efforts to lose weight elsewhere.

Cortisol and Insulin Resistance: A Vicious Cycle

One of the key ways cortisol contributes to belly fat is through its impact on **insulin**, the hormone responsible for regulating blood sugar levels. When cortisol is chronically elevated, it makes your cells less sensitive to insulin, leading to **insulin resistance**. This means that glucose stays in your bloodstream longer, prompting your body to produce more insulin in an effort to regulate your blood sugar.

Here's how this affects belly fat:

- **Insulin resistance promotes fat storage**: When your body produces more insulin, it also promotes fat storage, particularly in the belly. This is because insulin encourages your body to store excess glucose as fat, and the abdominal area is particularly prone to this kind of fat storage.

- **Blood sugar fluctuations**: Insulin resistance can cause blood sugar levels to spike and crash, leading to cravings for sugary and high-fat foods. This, combined with cortisol's effects on hunger hormones, can lead to overeating and further fat accumulation in the belly area.

Stress Eating and Cortisol

Another key factor that links cortisol to belly fat is its effect on **appetite and cravings**. When your cortisol levels are elevated, you're more likely to crave high-calorie, high-fat foods—comfort foods that provide quick energy. This is because cortisol stimulates the release of **ghrelin**, the hormone responsible for hunger, and can suppress **leptin**, the hormone that signals fullness.

This combination makes stress eating a real issue, especially when you're reaching for sugary snacks or processed foods to cope with your stress. Unfortunately, these foods are easily converted into fat, which often gets stored in your abdominal area due to cortisol's fat-storing tendencies.

The Role of Inflammation in Belly Fat Accumulation

Chronic stress not only raises cortisol levels but also increases **inflammation** in your body. Visceral fat, the type of fat that accumulates around your organs in the belly, is particularly inflammatory. This creates a cycle where:

- **Elevated cortisol leads to more belly fat**, which increases inflammation.
- **Increased inflammation raises cortisol levels**, creating a vicious cycle of stress and fat storage.

This inflammatory response is dangerous because it doesn't just contribute to weight gain. It's also associated with a higher risk of conditions like heart disease, type 2 diabetes, and metabolic syndrome, making belly fat not just a cosmetic issue but a serious health concern.

How Elevated Cortisol Impacts Exercise Efforts

If you've been exercising regularly but find that your belly fat isn't budging, cortisol may again be playing a role. When cortisol is elevated, your body prefers to burn **glucose** for energy rather than **fat**. This means that even if you're exercising, your body may not be burning fat as efficiently as it could be.

- **Over-exercising can increase cortisol**: Ironically, high-intensity exercise can sometimes raise cortisol levels even further, especially if you're already stressed. This is why balance is key. Overdoing it in the gym can work against your fat loss efforts if it's contributing to more stress in your body.
- **Restorative exercise**: Incorporating stress-reducing exercises like yoga, walking, or gentle stretching can help lower cortisol levels and promote fat burning. These types of movement signal to your body that it's safe, allowing cortisol levels to decrease and making fat loss, especially in the belly, more achievable.

Understanding the link between cortisol and belly fat is crucial for finding a sustainable solution to weight loss. It's not just about cutting calories or exercising more—it's about managing your stress and bringing cortisol back into balance. When you do, your body will respond more positively to the healthy changes you're making, and that stubborn belly fat will finally start to shift.

How Cortisol Sabotages Your Diet and Weight Loss Efforts

If you've ever felt like you're doing everything right—eating healthy, cutting calories, exercising regularly—yet you're still not seeing the weight loss results you expected, cortisol might be the hidden culprit. As your body's primary stress hormone, cortisol is designed to help you navigate stressful situations by providing the energy and focus you need to survive. However, when cortisol remains elevated over long periods, it can work against you, sabotaging your weight loss efforts in ways that aren't immediately obvious.

How Cortisol Affects Your Metabolism

One of the primary ways cortisol disrupts weight loss is by slowing down your **metabolism**. When you're under stress, cortisol signals your body to hold onto fat, especially in the abdominal area, in preparation for the perceived threat. This was helpful for our ancestors who needed to store energy during times of famine or danger, but in modern life, it works against your efforts to lose weight.

Here's how it plays out:

- **Energy conservation mode**: Chronically elevated cortisol signals to your body that it needs to conserve energy. As a result, your body becomes more efficient at storing calories as fat, particularly around your midsection.

- **Muscle breakdown**: Cortisol breaks down muscle tissue to release amino acids, which are then converted into glucose for quick energy. While this is useful in short-term emergencies, over time, it leads to a reduction in lean muscle mass. Since muscle is metabolically active tissue, less muscle means a slower metabolism, making it harder to burn calories, even at rest.

This combination of increased fat storage and reduced muscle mass creates a situation where your body is more likely to gain weight than lose it, despite your efforts to eat well and stay active.

Cortisol and Cravings

Cortisol has a direct impact on your **appetite** and the types of foods you crave, especially during periods of stress. When cortisol levels are elevated, your body craves high-calorie, high-sugar foods that provide a quick energy boost. These cravings are driven by the brain's need for fast fuel to cope with perceived threats, but in everyday life, this often leads to unhealthy eating patterns.

- **Craving sugar and fat**: Cortisol triggers the release of glucose into your bloodstream to provide energy, but when that energy isn't used (as is often the case with emotional or mental stress), you end up storing the excess glucose as fat. At the same time, cortisol makes you crave foods that will quickly replenish your blood sugar, particularly those high in sugar and fat.

- **Emotional eating**: When you're stressed, you're more likely to eat for emotional reasons rather than hunger. Cortisol increases levels of **ghrelin**, the "hunger hormone," while reducing **leptin**, the hormone that tells you when you're full. This hormonal imbalance can make it difficult to stop eating once you've started, leading to overeating and weight gain.

Blood Sugar Imbalances and Cortisol

Cortisol plays a critical role in regulating **blood sugar levels**, and this has a significant impact on weight loss. Under normal circumstances, cortisol helps maintain steady blood sugar levels, but when stress is chronic, cortisol disrupts this balance.

- **Insulin resistance**: Elevated cortisol levels can lead to insulin resistance, a condition in which your cells no longer respond effectively to insulin. As a result, glucose remains in your bloodstream for longer periods, forcing your body to produce more insulin to compensate. This excess insulin promotes fat storage, particularly in the belly, and makes it harder to lose weight.

- **Energy crashes**: Chronic stress and elevated cortisol can cause your blood sugar to spike and then crash, leaving you feeling fatigued and craving more sugar to restore your energy. This cycle of blood sugar highs and lows leads to overeating, further complicating your weight loss efforts.

The Impact of Cortisol on Exercise

You may think that increasing your physical activity would counteract the effects of cortisol on your weight, but it's not that simple. While exercise is essential for weight loss and overall health, the wrong type of exercise can actually increase cortisol levels, making it harder to shed pounds.

- **High-intensity workouts**: Intense exercise, especially when done for long durations or without proper recovery, can elevate cortisol levels. While your body needs a temporary cortisol spike during exercise to fuel your muscles, prolonged elevated cortisol after your workout can hinder fat loss. This is especially true if you're already dealing with high stress in other areas of your life.
- **Overtraining**: Too much exercise without adequate rest can put your body under chronic stress, leading to more cortisol production. Instead of helping you lose weight, overtraining can actually cause your body to hold onto fat, especially in the abdominal area.

Balancing your exercise routine with stress-reducing activities like yoga, walking, or stretching can help lower cortisol levels and support weight loss.

Cortisol and Sleep Disruption

One of the most frustrating ways cortisol interferes with weight loss is by disrupting your **sleep**. Normally, cortisol follows a natural rhythm, peaking in the morning to wake you up and tapering off throughout the day to help you relax and prepare for sleep. However, chronic stress can throw this rhythm out of balance, keeping cortisol levels elevated at night.

- **Difficulty falling asleep**: Elevated cortisol can make it hard to wind down at night, leading to difficulty falling asleep or staying asleep. Poor sleep directly impacts your ability to lose weight, as sleep deprivation increases ghrelin (hunger hormone) and decreases leptin (fullness hormone), making you more likely to overeat the next day.
- **Fatigue and cravings**: Lack of sleep also leaves you feeling fatigued during the day, which can lead to increased cravings for sugary or high-fat foods as your body seeks quick sources of energy.

Breaking the Cycle

To successfully lose weight, managing your cortisol levels is just as important as what you eat and how much you exercise. By reducing stress, prioritizing sleep, and balancing your hormones, you can stop cortisol from sabotaging your weight loss efforts and finally achieve the results you're working so hard for.

The Importance of Managing Cortisol for Long-Term Weight Control

If you're serious about achieving long-term weight control, managing cortisol is just as crucial as your diet and exercise routine. While many weight loss strategies focus solely on cutting calories and increasing physical activity, they often overlook how stress and cortisol levels influence fat storage, metabolism, and cravings. The truth is, if your cortisol remains chronically elevated, your body will resist weight loss efforts, no matter how disciplined you are with food and exercise. Understanding the role cortisol plays and learning how to manage it effectively is key to achieving lasting results.

Cortisol's Role in Fat Storage and Weight Retention

Cortisol is intricately connected to how your body stores fat, especially in the abdominal area. Elevated cortisol levels, whether caused by emotional stress, physical overexertion, or even lack of sleep, signal your body to prioritize storing energy as fat. This is because cortisol's primary function is to help you survive stressful situations by ensuring that you have enough energy reserves in case of prolonged challenges.

Here's how cortisol leads to long-term fat storage:

- **Fat deposition in the belly**: When cortisol is chronically elevated, your body prefers to store fat around your midsection, known as visceral fat. This type of fat is not only stubborn and harder to lose, but it also increases your risk for metabolic diseases like diabetes and heart disease.
- **Breaking down muscle**: High cortisol levels lead to muscle breakdown, which further slows your metabolism. Since muscle burns more calories at rest than fat, losing muscle mass makes it even harder to keep weight off in the long term.
- **Insulin resistance**: Chronically high cortisol disrupts your body's insulin response, making it difficult to regulate blood sugar levels. This leads to insulin resistance, where your body stores excess sugar as fat and makes it nearly impossible to shed pounds, especially in the abdominal area.

Managing Cortisol for Long-Term Weight Stability

To achieve sustainable weight loss, you need to bring cortisol levels back into balance. This doesn't mean eliminating stress completely—after all, some stress is inevitable—but it does mean learning how to manage it effectively so that it doesn't wreak havoc on your weight and health. Here are key strategies to consider:

- **Prioritize sleep**: Lack of sleep is one of the biggest contributors to elevated cortisol levels. When you don't get enough rest, your body stays in a state of heightened stress, causing cortisol to spike. This not only leads to weight gain but also makes it harder to lose fat, even if you're sticking to a healthy diet and exercise routine.
- *Actionable tip:* Aim for 7-9 hours of quality sleep each night. Create a calming bedtime routine and avoid screens or caffeine in the hours leading up to sleep to encourage deeper rest.
- **Eat a cortisol-friendly diet**: Your diet plays a massive role in managing cortisol. Eating a balanced diet that stabilizes blood sugar can help keep cortisol in check and support your weight loss goals.
- *Focus on:* Lean proteins, whole grains, fiber-rich vegetables, and healthy fats like Omega-3s, which help lower cortisol levels and reduce inflammation in the body. Avoid processed sugars, caffeine, and alcohol, which can cause spikes in blood sugar and cortisol.
- **Incorporate restorative exercise**: While intense workouts can be great for burning calories, they can also increase cortisol levels if overdone. High-intensity training without adequate recovery can lead to overtraining, which causes your body to produce more cortisol rather than burn fat.
- *Actionable tip:* Balance high-intensity workouts with restorative exercises like yoga, walking, or swimming. These activities reduce stress and promote fat loss by calming your nervous system and allowing cortisol levels to decrease naturally.

The Emotional Component of Cortisol and Weight

Chronic stress, whether from work, family life, or internal pressures, leads to emotional eating—a key factor in weight gain. When cortisol is elevated, your brain craves high-calorie, comfort foods as a quick source of energy. This biological drive makes it difficult to resist cravings, leading to overeating and further weight retention.

Managing cortisol means addressing the emotional aspects of stress. **Mindfulness practices** such as meditation, deep breathing, and journaling can help you become more aware of your stress triggers and teach you how to respond without reaching for food. Reducing emotional stress can break the cycle of cortisol-driven overeating and help you regain control over your eating habits.

Maintaining Cortisol Balance for Long-Term Success

Once you've worked to lower your cortisol levels, it's crucial to maintain that balance for sustained weight control. This requires ongoing commitment to stress management practices, regular sleep, and a balanced lifestyle that supports both your mental and physical health. Cortisol is dynamic, meaning it can easily become elevated again if you allow stress to dominate your life.

- **Stress reduction habits**: Establish daily habits that keep stress in check, such as taking breaks during the workday, spending time outdoors, or practicing gratitude. Small, consistent efforts to reduce stress will help you maintain lower cortisol levels, making it easier to keep the weight off in the long term.

- **Consistency is key**: Long-term weight management requires consistency, not perfection. Prioritizing habits that reduce cortisol and create balance in your body will result in sustainable weight control without drastic or extreme measures.

By focusing on managing cortisol alongside traditional diet and exercise strategies, you're not just losing weight temporarily—you're setting yourself up for a lifetime of healthier living. Bringing cortisol back into balance will help you regain control over your body, allowing you to achieve the long-term results you've been striving for.

CHAPTER 3

Breaking the Cycle of Fatigue and Stress

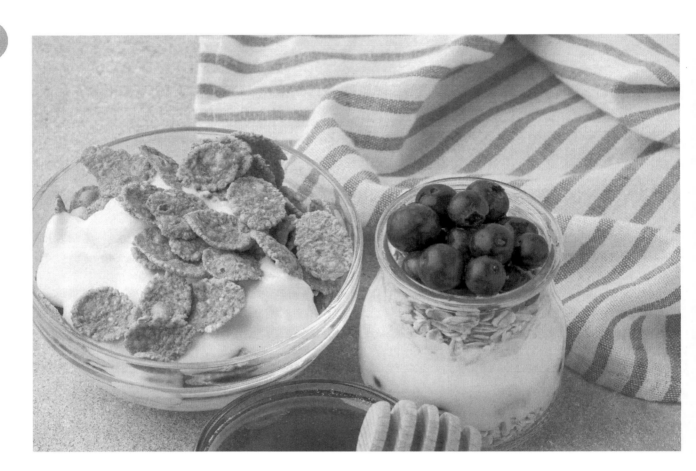

Why You Feel Tired All the Time: The Cortisol Trap

If you find yourself constantly feeling exhausted, even after what should have been a full night of rest, you're not alone. For many women, this persistent fatigue is not just the result of a busy life—it's a direct consequence of being stuck in the **cortisol trap**. Cortisol, your body's primary stress hormone, is supposed to help you manage immediate challenges and restore balance. However, when stress becomes chronic, elevated cortisol levels can sabotage your energy, leaving you feeling drained day after day. Understanding how this happens is the first step in breaking free from this cycle of fatigue and stress.

The Cortisol Rhythm: What's Supposed to Happen?

Under normal circumstances, cortisol follows a **diurnal rhythm**. It peaks in the morning, giving you the boost you need to wake up and tackle the day, and gradually declines throughout the afternoon and evening, preparing your body for rest. This natural ebb and flow of cortisol is essential for maintaining energy levels, supporting metabolism, and managing stress.

Here's how it should work:

- **Morning peak**: Cortisol levels rise in the early hours of the morning, helping you feel alert and awake.
- **Daytime decline**: Throughout the day, cortisol slowly decreases, ensuring that you have steady energy without feeling overstimulated.
- **Evening low**: By nighttime, cortisol levels should be low, signaling to your body that it's time to wind down and sleep.

When cortisol follows this healthy rhythm, your energy is balanced, and you wake up feeling refreshed. But when stress becomes a constant part of your life, this rhythm is thrown off balance, leading to a cascade of problems, including persistent fatigue.

The Cortisol Trap: Chronic Stress and Energy Depletion

The **cortisol trap** happens when your body is exposed to ongoing stress, causing cortisol levels to remain elevated or dysregulated. Instead of following its normal rhythm, cortisol may spike at the wrong times or stay elevated throughout the day, leaving you stuck in a state of chronic stress and fatigue.

- **Cortisol overload**: When cortisol levels are consistently high, your body is in a perpetual state of fight-or-flight mode. This drains your energy reserves because cortisol demands constant glucose production to keep you alert. Over time, this state of heightened stress exhausts your body, leading to a sense of constant tiredness, even if you're not physically exerting yourself.
- **HPA axis dysregulation**: Chronic stress impacts the **hypothalamic-pituitary-adrenal (HPA) axis**, which regulates cortisol production. When the HPA axis becomes overworked, it struggles to maintain balance. This leads to irregular cortisol levels, meaning you might experience a cortisol spike late in the day, disrupting your sleep and leaving you tired the next morning.
- **Energy crashes**: Cortisol disrupts blood sugar regulation, leading to peaks and crashes in energy. When your body releases too much glucose into the bloodstream in response to cortisol, it can lead to energy highs followed by sharp crashes, causing fatigue and cravings for quick fixes like sugar and caffeine.

How Cortisol Impacts Sleep

Cortisol is supposed to be low at night, allowing melatonin—the hormone that regulates sleep—to do its job. However, elevated cortisol levels can keep your body in a heightened state of alertness, making it difficult to fall asleep, stay asleep, or get deep, restorative rest.

- **Delayed sleep onset**: High cortisol in the evening can make it hard to wind down, leaving you lying in bed, mind racing, long after you've turned out the lights.
- **Frequent wake-ups**: Even if you manage to fall asleep, elevated cortisol can cause you to wake up throughout the night or wake up too early in the morning. This disrupts the deep sleep cycles that are crucial for energy restoration.

- **Poor sleep quality**: Elevated cortisol interferes with your ability to enter deep sleep stages, meaning your sleep may be shallow and unrefreshing. As a result, you wake up feeling tired, regardless of how many hours you've spent in bed.

The Fatigue-Stress Cycle

What makes the cortisol trap so difficult to escape is that **fatigue and stress feed into each other**, creating a vicious cycle that's hard to break. Here's how the cycle typically works:

1. **Stress triggers cortisol**: You experience stress—whether it's from work, family, or other pressures—and your body releases cortisol in response.
2. **Cortisol disrupts sleep**: Elevated cortisol makes it difficult to sleep, leading to poor-quality rest.
3. **Fatigue sets in**: As your sleep suffers, so does your energy. You wake up feeling exhausted and rely on stimulants like caffeine to get through the day.
4. **More stress, more cortisol**: The fatigue makes it harder to cope with stress, leading to even more cortisol production. And the cycle continues.

This cycle of stress and fatigue is self-perpetuating: the more stressed you are, the more tired you feel; the more tired you feel, the harder it is to manage stress. Over time, this cycle leads to **adrenal fatigue**, where your adrenal glands become depleted from overproducing cortisol. At this point, your energy levels crash, and even small tasks feel overwhelming.

The Consequences of Chronic Fatigue

Left unchecked, the cortisol trap can lead to a range of health problems that extend beyond just feeling tired. Chronic fatigue caused by elevated cortisol is linked to:

- **Weakened immune system**: High cortisol levels suppress your immune function, making you more susceptible to infections and illnesses.
- **Weight gain**: Persistent fatigue often leads to cravings for sugary and high-fat foods, which provide quick energy but contribute to weight gain, especially in the abdominal area.
- **Mood imbalances**: Chronic fatigue and stress can lead to anxiety, irritability, and even depression as your body and mind struggle to cope with the constant pressure.
- **Hormonal disruptions**: Elevated cortisol affects other hormones like thyroid and reproductive hormones, leading to imbalances that further contribute to feelings of fatigue and low energy.

Recognizing the Signs of Cortisol-Driven Fatigue

If you're feeling tired all the time despite getting adequate rest, cortisol-driven fatigue might be to blame. Common signs that cortisol is behind your fatigue include:

- Waking up tired, even after a full night's sleep.
- Craving sugary or high-carb foods for quick energy boosts.
- Feeling "wired but tired"—exhausted yet unable to relax or fall asleep.
- Frequent mood swings or irritability, especially during high-stress periods.
- Mid-afternoon energy crashes that leave you reaching for caffeine or sweets.

By understanding how cortisol disrupts your energy levels, you can begin to take the necessary steps to break free from this cycle and reclaim your vitality.

How Stress Disrupts Your Sleep and Lowers Your Energy

If you've ever spent a sleepless night worrying about the stresses of the day, you've experienced firsthand how stress can disrupt your sleep. What you may not realize is that even low-level, ongoing stress can have a profound impact on the quality of your sleep and, in turn, drain your energy. This disruption isn't just about a restless night here and there—it's a cycle that gradually chips away at your ability to recover, leaving you feeling fatigued no matter how much time you spend in bed.

The Cortisol-Sleep Connection

Cortisol, your body's main stress hormone, follows a natural rhythm that is closely linked to your sleep-wake cycle. Under ideal conditions, cortisol peaks in the morning to help wake you up and gradually declines throughout the day, reaching its lowest point at night when melatonin, the sleep hormone, takes over. This balance is crucial for falling asleep and staying asleep.

When you're under stress, however, this delicate balance is disrupted. Instead of decreasing in the evening, cortisol levels can remain elevated, preventing your body from winding down and making it harder to fall asleep.

- **Delayed sleep onset**: When cortisol levels are high in the evening, your mind stays alert, racing with thoughts about the day's challenges or tomorrow's tasks. This makes it difficult to relax enough to fall asleep, leaving you tossing and turning in bed.

- **Nighttime wake-ups**: Even if you do manage to fall asleep, elevated cortisol can cause you to wake up frequently throughout the night, preventing you from reaching the deeper, restorative stages of sleep your body needs to recover.

- **Morning grogginess**: High cortisol levels in the evening can push your natural rhythm out of sync, making it harder to wake up feeling refreshed. You may feel groggy or experience that "foggy" sensation, even if you technically got enough hours of sleep.

The Role of Adrenaline and the Fight-or-Flight Response

Stress doesn't just elevate cortisol—it also triggers the **fight-or-flight response**, which involves the release of adrenaline. Adrenaline is another hormone designed to help you react quickly in times of danger by increasing your heart rate, raising your blood pressure, and pumping more blood to your muscles.

While these effects are useful in a life-threatening situation, they are counterproductive when you're trying to rest. If your body is flooded with adrenaline due to stress, it becomes incredibly difficult to relax. Your body remains in a heightened state of alertness, making restful sleep almost impossible.

- **Increased heart rate**: Adrenaline keeps your heart rate elevated, which makes it harder for your body to reach the calm, steady state required for sleep.

- **Restlessness**: Adrenaline can cause physical restlessness, making it difficult to get comfortable or stay still during the night.

How Stress Affects Sleep Quality

Even if stress doesn't prevent you from falling asleep, it can still interfere with the **quality** of your sleep. High cortisol levels disrupt the normal progression of sleep stages, preventing you from reaching the deep sleep phases that are essential for physical and mental recovery.

- **REM sleep disruption**: Stress can interfere with **REM sleep**, the stage of sleep associated with dreaming and emotional processing. Without enough REM sleep, your brain doesn't get the chance to process stress and emotions from the day, leading to increased anxiety and irritability the next day.
- **Lack of deep sleep**: Deep sleep, also known as **slow-wave sleep**, is when your body repairs tissues, builds muscle, and strengthens your immune system. Chronic stress reduces the amount of time you spend in deep sleep, leaving your body less equipped to recover and restore itself.

The Impact on Energy Levels

When stress disrupts your sleep, it has a direct impact on your energy levels during the day. Sleep is your body's way of recharging, and without quality sleep, you start the day with less energy in reserve. Over time, this leads to **chronic fatigue**, where you feel tired all the time, even if you're spending enough hours in bed.

- **Daytime fatigue**: Without restorative sleep, your body struggles to keep up with daily demands. You may feel sluggish, unmotivated, or like you're constantly running on empty.
- **Reduced cognitive function**: Lack of sleep impairs your cognitive abilities, making it harder to concentrate, stay focused, and think clearly. This mental fog can leave you feeling even more stressed, as you struggle to keep up with your responsibilities.
- **Weakened immune system**: Prolonged sleep disruption weakens your immune system, making you more susceptible to illnesses and infections. This further drains your energy, as your body uses its limited resources to fight off illness rather than keep you energized.

The Vicious Cycle of Stress, Sleep, and Energy

One of the most challenging aspects of stress-related sleep disruption is the **vicious cycle** it creates. Poor sleep leads to low energy, which makes it harder to manage stress. As your stress levels rise, cortisol increases, further disrupting your sleep and perpetuating the cycle.

Here's how the cycle typically plays out:

1. **Stress triggers elevated cortisol levels**, which make it harder to fall asleep.
2. **Sleep disruption leads to poor-quality sleep**, preventing your body from fully recovering.
3. **Fatigue sets in**, leaving you feeling drained and unable to cope with stress effectively.
4. **Increased stress from fatigue** causes cortisol levels to rise even further, leading to more sleep disruption.

Breaking this cycle requires addressing both the stress and the sleep disruption simultaneously. By managing stress during the day, you can lower cortisol levels in the evening, making it easier to fall asleep and stay asleep. Once your sleep improves, your energy levels will begin to rebound, making it easier to manage stress and maintain a healthy sleep cycle.

If stress is disrupting your sleep, you might notice several telltale signs:

- **Difficulty falling asleep**, even when you feel tired.
- **Waking up frequently** during the night, often with a racing mind.
- **Feeling tired or groggy** in the morning, despite spending enough time in bed.
- **Mid-afternoon energy crashes**, leaving you feeling drained and craving caffeine or sugar for a quick energy boost.

By identifying these patterns, you can start taking steps to manage your stress, improve your sleep, and restore your energy levels.

Actionable Strategies to Break Free from the Stress-Fatigue Cycle

Breaking free from the stress-fatigue cycle requires a holistic approach that targets both the physical and mental aspects of stress. It's not enough to simply address one area—you need to create a routine that tackles stress management, restores energy, and helps your body recover from the effects of chronic cortisol elevation. Below are practical, actionable strategies to help you regain your vitality and escape the cycle of stress and fatigue.

1.   Prioritize Quality Sleep

One of the most effective ways to lower cortisol levels and restore energy is by improving your sleep. When you're well-rested, your body can better regulate cortisol, allowing you to manage stress more effectively. To achieve this, you need to focus on both the quantity and quality of your sleep.

- **Establish a bedtime routine**: Create a consistent sleep schedule by going to bed and waking up at the same time every day, even on weekends. This helps regulate your body's internal clock and supports the natural cortisol rhythm.
- **Limit screen time before bed**: The blue light emitted by screens suppresses melatonin, the hormone that helps you sleep. Avoid screens at least one hour before bedtime to allow your body to wind down naturally.
- **Create a calming environment**: Your bedroom should be a sanctuary for sleep. Keep it dark, quiet, and cool, and consider using white noise or earplugs to block out distractions.

2.   Practice Mindfulness and Stress Reduction Techniques

Since stress is the primary driver of cortisol, incorporating stress-reducing practices into your daily routine is essential for breaking the cycle of fatigue. These techniques help calm the mind, lower cortisol, and promote a sense of relaxation that supports both mental and physical recovery.

- **Deep breathing exercises**: Deep, controlled breathing activates the parasympathetic nervous system, which helps to lower cortisol and reduce the fight-or-flight response. Try the **4-7-8 breathing technique**: inhale for four seconds, hold for seven, and exhale for eight. This can be done anytime you feel stressed.
- **Meditation**: Regular meditation helps quiet the mind and lower cortisol levels. Even just 10 minutes a day of mindfulness meditation can make a significant difference in how your body handles stress.
- **Progressive muscle relaxation**: This technique involves tensing and then slowly relaxing each

muscle group in your body. It helps release physical tension while signaling to your brain that it's time to relax, reducing cortisol levels.

3. Eat a Cortisol-Balancing Diet

Your diet plays a crucial role in regulating cortisol levels. Certain foods can either spike cortisol or help keep it in check, so it's important to be mindful of what you're eating. A cortisol-friendly diet focuses on stabilizing blood sugar levels and reducing inflammation.

- **Eat whole foods**: Prioritize whole, unprocessed foods that provide steady energy and prevent blood sugar spikes. Foods like leafy greens, nuts, seeds, lean proteins, and healthy fats (like those found in avocados and fatty fish) are excellent for balancing cortisol.

- **Avoid sugar and refined carbs**: These cause rapid spikes in blood sugar, followed by crashes that increase cortisol. Instead, choose complex carbohydrates like quinoa, brown rice, or sweet potatoes, which provide more stable energy.

- **Stay hydrated**: Dehydration can lead to an increase in cortisol levels. Make sure you're drinking enough water throughout the day—about 8-10 glasses is a good target. Herbal teas like chamomile or peppermint can also help soothe your body and mind.

4. Incorporate Low-Impact, Restorative Movement

While exercise is an important part of staying healthy, too much high-intensity activity can actually raise cortisol levels, especially if you're already stressed. Incorporating gentle, restorative movements into your routine can help you stay active while lowering cortisol and relieving stress.

- **Walking**: A daily 20-30 minute walk, particularly in nature, can significantly lower cortisol levels. Walking also boosts endorphins, the body's natural feel-good hormones, which help counteract stress.

- **Yoga**: Gentle yoga practices, particularly those that focus on breathing and relaxation, are incredibly effective for lowering cortisol. Poses that emphasize deep stretching and slow movement help activate the parasympathetic nervous system, encouraging relaxation.

- **Stretching**: A simple stretching routine before bed can help release physical tension and signal to your body that it's time to relax and recover.

5. Manage Your Workload and Set Boundaries

One of the most common sources of stress is an overwhelming workload and the pressure to always be "on." Learning to manage your workload and set healthy boundaries is essential for reducing stress and keeping cortisol levels in check.

- **Set realistic goals**: Break large tasks into smaller, manageable steps and set realistic deadlines. This reduces the feeling of being overwhelmed and helps prevent the cortisol spike that comes with trying to do too much at once.

- **Learn to say no**: If you're someone who feels obligated to say yes to every request, it's time to set boundaries. Politely declining tasks that exceed your capacity is essential for maintaining your mental health and reducing stress.

- **Take regular breaks**: Incorporate short breaks throughout your day to allow your mind and body to rest. Even just five minutes of stepping away from your desk, stretching, or doing a quick breathing exercise can help lower cortisol and restore energy.

6. Make Time for Joyful Activities

Engaging in activities that bring you joy and relaxation is one of the best ways to lower cortisol levels and break free from the stress-fatigue cycle. These activities can be simple and don't have to take up a lot of time, but they should be things that genuinely bring you happiness.

- **Hobbies**: Whether it's reading, gardening, painting, or cooking, engaging in hobbies that you enjoy can lower cortisol and provide a mental escape from stress.
- **Social connection**: Spending time with loved ones, even for short periods, can lower cortisol and improve your mood. Socializing releases oxytocin, a hormone that counteracts the effects of stress and helps you feel connected and supported.
- **Laughter**: Something as simple as watching a funny movie or spending time with someone who makes you laugh can lower cortisol and boost your overall sense of well-being.

By implementing these strategies into your daily routine, you can break the cycle of stress and fatigue, lower cortisol levels, and restore your energy. Taking small, consistent steps toward managing stress and supporting your body will lead to long-lasting improvements in your health and vitality.

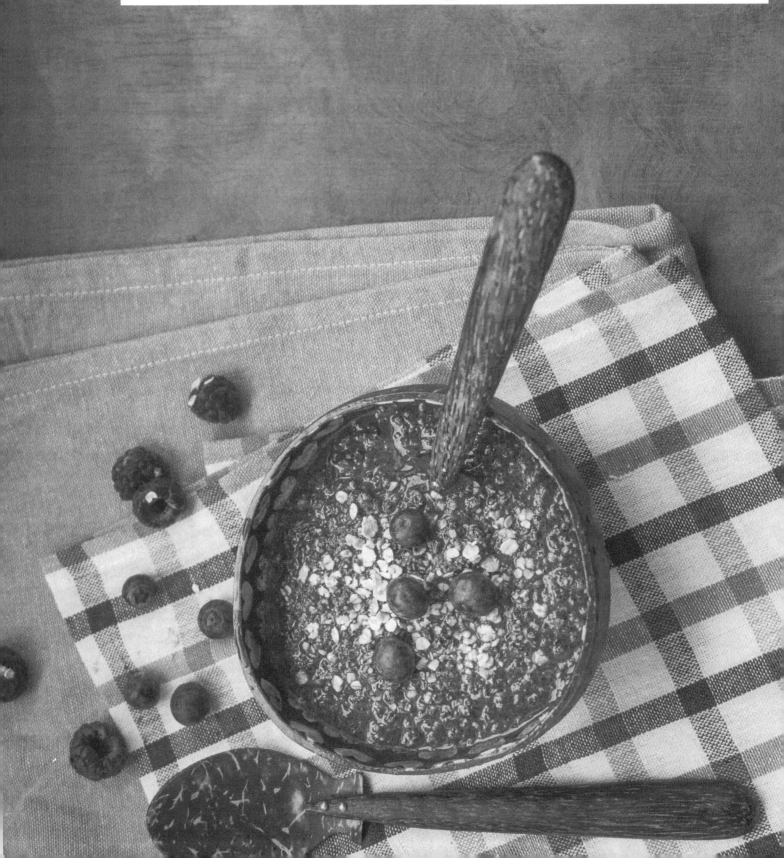

PART 2

75 Recipes for Balancing Cortisol

CHAPTER 4

Breakfast Recipes

Avocado and Spinach Scramble

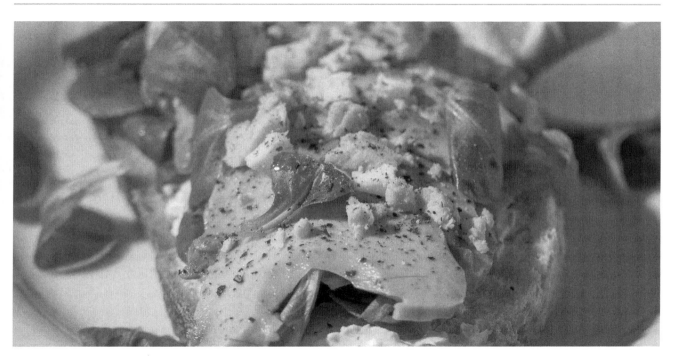

Preparation Time: 5 minutes   **Cooking Time:** 10 minutes   **Servings:** 2

INGREDIENTS:

- 2 eggs
- 1 ripe avocado, diced
- 1 cup fresh spinach, chopped
- 1 tbsp olive oil
- Salt and pepper to taste
- Optional: Feta cheese (omit for dairy-free)

PREPARATION:

1. Heat olive oil in a pan over medium heat.
2. Add spinach and sauté until wilted, about 2 minutes.
3. In a bowl, whisk eggs with salt and pepper. Pour the eggs over the spinach and scramble until cooked through.
4. Add diced avocado and mix gently.
5. Serve hot, with optional feta cheese on top.

Nutritional Information: Calories: 250; Carbohydrates: 7g; Protein: 10g; Fat: 22g; Fiber: 6g; Vitamins: A, C, K; Potassium: 700mg; Sodium: 140mg; Sugar: 1g.

Chia Seed Pudding with Berries

Preparation Time: 5 minutes + overnight chilling

Cooking Time: 0 minutes

Servings: 2

INGREDIENTS:

- 1/4 cup chia seeds
- 1 cup almond milk (or any non-dairy milk)
- 1 tbsp maple syrup
- 1/2 tsp vanilla extract
- 1/2 cup mixed berries

PREPARATION:

1. In a bowl, combine chia seeds, almond milk, maple syrup, and vanilla extract. Stir well.
2. Let sit for 5 minutes, then stir again to prevent clumping.
3. Cover and refrigerate overnight.
4. In the morning, top with mixed berries before serving.

Nutritional Information: Calories: 180; Carbohydrates: 24g; Protein: 5g; Fat: 9g; Fiber: 9g; Vitamins: C, K; Potassium: 200mg; Sodium: 50mg; Sugar: 12g.

Oatmeal with Pumpkin Seeds and Dried Cranberries

Preparation Time: 5 minutes

Cooking Time: 10 minutes

Servings: 1

INGREDIENTS:

- 1/2 cup rolled oats
- 1 cup water or almond milk
- 1 tbsp pumpkin seeds
- 1 tbsp dried cranberries
- 1 tsp cinnamon

PREPARATION:

1. Cook oats in water or almond milk over medium heat for 5-7 minutes until soft.
2. Stir in cinnamon.
3. Top with pumpkin seeds and dried cranberries before serving.

Nutritional Information: Calories: 220; Carbohydrates: 42g; Protein: 6g; Fat: 6g; Fiber: 6g; Vitamins: B6, E; Potassium: 200mg; Sodium: 50mg; Sugar: 12g.

Quinoa Porridge with Almonds and Blueberries

Preparation Time: 5 minutes   **Cooking Time:** 15 minutes   **Servings:** 2

INGREDIENTS:

- 1/2 cup quinoa
- 1 cup almond milk (or non-dairy milk)
- 1/2 tsp cinnamon
- 1 tbsp maple syrup
- 1/4 cup blueberries
- 2 tbsp sliced almonds

PREPARATION:

1. Rinse quinoa and place in a saucepan with almond milk. Bring to a boil.
2. Reduce heat to low and simmer for 15 minutes, until quinoa is tender.
3. Stir in cinnamon and maple syrup.
4. Serve in bowls, topped with blueberries and almonds.

Nutritional Information: Calories: 250; Carbohydrates: 38g; Protein: 8g; Fat: 8g; Fiber: 6g; Vitamins: C, E; Potassium: 300mg; Sodium: 50mg; Sugar: 8g.

Sweet Potato and Kale Breakfast Hash

Preparation Time: 10 minutes   **Cooking Time:** 20 minutes   **Servings:** 2

INGREDIENTS:

- 1 medium sweet potato, diced
- 1 cup fresh kale, chopped
- 1/2 onion, diced
- 2 eggs
- 1 tbsp olive oil
- Salt and pepper to taste

PREPARATION:

1. Heat olive oil in a skillet over medium heat. Add diced sweet potatoes and onions. Cook for 10-12 minutes until tender.
2. Add kale and sauté for another 2-3 minutes until wilted.
3. In a separate pan, cook the eggs to your preference (scrambled or sunny-side-up).
4. Serve the sweet potato and kale mixture with the eggs on top.

Nutritional Information: Calories: 280; Carbohydrates: 26g; Protein: 12g; Fat: 16g; Fiber: 7g; Vitamins: A, C, K; Potassium: 800mg; Sodium: 100mg; Sugar: 6g.

Greek Yogurt with Flaxseeds and Fresh Strawberries

Preparation Time: 5 minutes   **Cooking Time:** 0 minutes   **Servings:** 1

INGREDIENTS:

- 1/2 cup Greek yogurt (dairy-free alternative: coconut yogurt)
- 1 tbsp ground flaxseeds
- 1/4 cup fresh strawberries, sliced
- 1 tsp honey or maple syrup

PREPARATION:

1. Place the Greek yogurt in a bowl.
2. Top with flaxseeds, sliced strawberries, and honey.
3. Stir gently before eating.

Nutritional Information: Calories: 150; Carbohydrates: 14g; Protein: 10g; Fat: 6g; Fiber: 4g; Vitamins: C, K; Potassium: 250mg; Sodium: 50mg; Sugar: 10g.

Steel-Cut Oats with Walnuts and Cinnamon

Preparation Time: 5 minutes   **Cooking Time:** 20 minutes   **Servings:** 2

INGREDIENTS:

- 1/2 cup steel-cut oats
- 2 cups water
- 1/4 cup walnuts, chopped
- 1 tsp cinnamon
- 1 tbsp maple syrup

PREPARATION:

1. Bring water to a boil, add steel-cut oats.
2. Reduce heat and simmer for 20 minutes until oats are tender.
3. Stir in cinnamon and maple syrup.
4. Serve topped with chopped walnuts.

Nutritional Information: Calories: 240; Carbohydrates: 38g; Protein: 6g; Fat: 10g; Fiber: 5g; Vitamins: B6, E; Potassium: 300mg; Sodium: 10mg; Sugar: 8g.

Almond Butter and Banana Smoothie

Preparation Time: 5 minutes   **Cooking Time:** 0 minutes   **Servings:** 1

INGREDIENTS:

- 1 banana
- 1 tbsp almond butter
- 1 cup almond milk
- 1 tbsp chia seeds
- Ice cubes

PREPARATION:

1. Combine all ingredients in a blender.
2. Blend until smooth.
3. Serve immediately.

Nutritional Information: Calories: 280; Carbohydrates: 35g; Protein: 7g; Fat: 12g; Fiber: 6g; Vitamins: C, B6; Potassium: 450mg; Sodium: 60mg; Sugar: 18g.

Scrambled Tofu with Spinach and Mushrooms

Preparation Time: 5 minutes   **Cooking Time:** 10 minutes   **Servings:** 2

INGREDIENTS:

- 200g firm tofu, crumbled
- 1 cup fresh spinach, chopped
- 1/2 cup mushrooms, sliced
- 1 tbsp olive oil
- 1/2 tsp turmeric
- Salt and pepper to taste

PREPARATION:

1. Heat olive oil in a skillet over medium heat. Add mushrooms and cook for 5 minutes.
2. Add spinach and cook for another 2 minutes until wilted.
3. Stir in crumbled tofu, turmeric, salt, and pepper. Cook for another 3-5 minutes.
4. Serve hot.

Nutritional Information: Calories: 220; Carbohydrates: 8g; Protein: 18g; Fat: 14g; Fiber: 4g; Vitamins: A, K; Potassium: 300mg; Sodium: 200mg; Sugar: 2g.

Overnight Oats with Chia Seeds and Almond Milk

Preparation Time: 5 minutes + overnight chilling   **Cooking Time:** 0 minutes   **Servings:** 1

INGREDIENTS:

- 1/2 cup rolled oats
- 1 tbsp chia seeds
- 1 cup almond milk
- 1/2 tsp vanilla extract
- 1 tbsp maple syrup

PREPARATION:

1. In a jar or bowl, combine oats, chia seeds, almond milk, vanilla extract, and maple syrup. Stir well.
2. Cover and refrigerate overnight.
3. In the morning, give it a stir and enjoy.

Nutritional Information: Calories: 220; Carbohydrates: 35g; Protein: 6g; Fat: 8g; Fiber: 8g; Vitamins: B6, E; Potassium: 250mg; Sodium: 60mg; Sugar: 10g.

Buckwheat Pancakes with Fresh Berries

Preparation Time: 10 minutes   **Cooking Time:** 10 minutes   **Servings:** 2

INGREDIENTS:

- 1/2 cup buckwheat flour
- 1/2 cup almond milk (or other non-dairy milk)
- 1 egg (or flaxseed egg for vegan option)
- 1 tsp baking powder
- 1 tbsp maple syrup
- Fresh berries for topping

PREPARATION:

1. In a bowl, mix buckwheat flour, baking powder, almond milk, egg, and maple syrup until smooth.
2. Heat a non-stick pan over medium heat and pour batter to form pancakes.
3. Cook for 2-3 minutes on each side until golden brown.
4. Serve with fresh berries on top.

Nutritional Information: Calories: 250; Carbohydrates: 36g; Protein: 8g; Fat: 7g; Fiber: 6g; Vitamins: B6, E; Potassium: 200mg; Sodium: 150mg; Sugar: 12g.

Green Smoothie with Kale, Avocado, and Flaxseeds

Preparation Time: 5 minutes   **Cooking Time:** 0 minutes   **Servings:** 1

INGREDIENTS:

- 1/2 avocado
- 1/2 cup fresh kale
- 1 tbsp flaxseeds
- 1 cup almond milk
- 1/2 banana

PREPARATION:

1. Combine all ingredients in a blender.
2. Blend until smooth.
3. Serve immediately.

Nutritional Information: Calories: 280; Carbohydrates: 24g; Protein: 5g; Fat: 18g; Fiber: 8g; Vitamins: A, C, E; Potassium: 500mg; Sodium: 60mg; Sugar: 10g.

Baked Eggs in Avocado Boats

Preparation Time: 5 minutes   **Cooking Time:** 15 minutes   **Servings:** 2

INGREDIENTS:

- 1 large avocado, halved and pitted
- 2 eggs
- Salt and pepper to taste
- Chopped chives for garnish

PREPARATION:

1. Preheat oven to 375°F (190°C).
2. Scoop out a bit of the avocado to make space for the egg.
3. Crack an egg into each avocado half.
4. Bake for 12-15 minutes until the egg whites are set.
5. Season with salt, pepper, and garnish with chives.

Nutritional Information: Calories: 300; Carbohydrates: 8g; Protein: 12g; Fat: 26g; Fiber: 10g; Vitamins: A, K; Potassium: 800mg; Sodium: 150mg; Sugar: 1g.

Coconut and Blueberry Smoothie Bowl

Preparation Time: 5 minutes   **Cooking Time:** 0 minutes   **Servings:** 1

INGREDIENTS:

- 1/2 cup coconut milk
- 1/2 cup frozen blueberries
- 1/4 cup coconut flakes
- 1 tbsp chia seeds
- 1 tbsp almond butter

PREPARATION:

1. Blend coconut milk, blueberries, and chia seeds until smooth.
2. Pour into a bowl and top with coconut flakes and almond butter.
3. Serve immediately.

Nutritional Information: Calories: 350; Carbohydrates: 24g; Protein: 7g; Fat: 28g; Fiber: 8g; Vitamins: C, E; Potassium: 200mg; Sodium: 50mg; Sugar: 10g.

Poached Eggs on Whole Grain Toast with Avocado

Preparation Time: 5 minutes   **Cooking Time:** 5 minutes   **Servings:** 2

INGREDIENTS:

- 2 eggs
- 2 slices whole grain bread
- 1 ripe avocado, mashed
- Salt and pepper to taste
- Chili flakes (optional)

PREPARATION:

1. Bring water to a simmer in a pot. Crack eggs into the water and poach for 3-4 minutes.
2. Toast the bread while the eggs cook.
3. Spread mashed avocado on the toasted bread.
4. Place the poached eggs on top of the avocado toast. Season with salt, pepper, and optional chili flakes.

Nutritional Information: Calories: 300; Carbohydrates: 30g; Protein: 12g; Fat: 18g; Fiber: 8g; Vitamins: A, K, B6; Potassium: 700mg; Sodium: 180mg; Sugar: 2g.

CHAPTER 5

Lunch Recipes

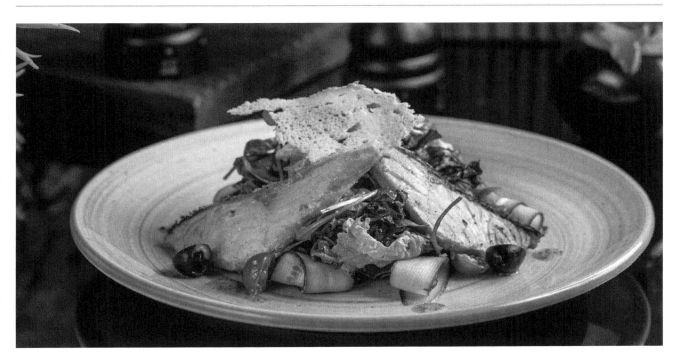

Grilled Salmon Salad with Spinach and Avocado

Preparation Time: 10 minutes   **Cooking Time:** 10 minutes   **Servings:** 2

INGREDIENTS:

- 2 salmon fillets
- 4 cups fresh spinach
- 1 avocado, sliced
- 1/2 cup cherry tomatoes, halved
- 2 tbsp olive oil
- 1 tbsp lemon juice
- Salt and pepper to taste

PREPARATION:

1. Season salmon with salt, pepper, and lemon juice. Grill for 4-5 minutes on each side.
2. In a large bowl, combine spinach, avocado, and cherry tomatoes.
3. Drizzle olive oil over the salad and toss gently.
4. Top with grilled salmon and serve immediately.

Nutritional Information: calories: 400; carbohydrates: 12g; protein: 34g; fat: 26g; fiber: 7g; vitamins: A, C, K; potassium: 950mg; sodium: 150mg; sugar: 3g.

Quinoa Salad with Chickpeas, Cucumber, and Feta

Preparation Time: 10 minutes   **Cooking Time:** 15 minutes   **Servings:** 2

INGREDIENTS:

- 1/2 cup quinoa, rinsed
- 1/2 cup canned chickpeas, drained
- 1/2 cucumber, diced
- 1/4 cup feta cheese (omit for dairy-free)
- 2 tbsp olive oil
- 1 tbsp lemon juice
- Salt and pepper to taste

PREPARATION:

1. Cook quinoa according to package instructions. Let it cool.
2. In a bowl, combine quinoa, chickpeas, cucumber, and feta.
3. Drizzle with olive oil and lemon juice, then toss gently.
4. Season with salt and pepper and serve.

Nutritional Information: calories: 350; carbohydrates: 38g; protein: 12g; fat: 18g; fiber: 6g; vitamins: C, K; potassium: 450mg; sodium: 300mg; sugar: 2g.

Farro Salad with Roasted Vegetables and Goat Cheese

Preparation Time: 15 minutes   **Cooking Time:** 30 minutes   **Servings:** 2

INGREDIENTS:

- 1/2 cup farro
- 1/2 cup roasted vegetables (zucchini, bell peppers)
- 1/4 cup goat cheese, crumbled (omit for dairy-free)
- 2 tbsp olive oil
- 1 tbsp balsamic vinegar
- Salt and pepper to taste

PREPARATION:

1. Cook farro according to package instructions. Let cool.
2. In a bowl, combine farro, roasted vegetables, and goat cheese.
3. Drizzle with olive oil and balsamic vinegar, then toss gently.
4. Season with salt and pepper and serve.

Nutritional Information: calories: 370; carbohydrates: 48g; protein: 14g; fat: 14g; fiber: 9g; vitamins: A, C, K; potassium: 600mg; sodium: 250mg; sugar: 6g.

Turkey Lettuce Wraps with Avocado and Salsa

Preparation Time: 10 minutes   **Cooking Time:** 10 minutes   **Servings:** 2

INGREDIENTS:

- 1/2 lb ground turkey
- 1 avocado, sliced
- 1/2 cup salsa
- 8 large lettuce leaves
- 1 tbsp olive oil
- Salt and pepper to taste

PREPARATION:

1. Heat olive oil in a skillet over medium heat and cook the ground turkey until fully cooked, about 8-10 minutes. Season with salt and pepper.
2. To assemble the wraps, place cooked turkey in lettuce leaves.
3. Top with avocado slices and salsa.
4. Serve immediately.

Nutritional Information: calories: 300; carbohydrates: 10g; protein: 28g; fat: 18g; fiber: 6g; vitamins: A, C, K; potassium: 700mg; sodium: 350mg; sugar: 2g.

Mediterranean Lentil Salad with Feta and Olive Oil

Preparation Time: 10 minutes   **Cooking Time:** 20 minutes   **Servings:** 2

INGREDIENTS:

- 1/2 cup green lentils
- 1/4 cup feta cheese (omit for dairy-free)
- 1/2 cucumber, diced
- 1/4 cup cherry tomatoes, halved
- 2 tbsp olive oil
- 1 tbsp red wine vinegar
- Salt and pepper to taste

PREPARATION:

1. Cook lentils according to package instructions. Drain and let cool.
2. In a bowl, combine lentils, cucumber, cherry tomatoes, and feta.
3. Drizzle with olive oil and red wine vinegar, then toss to combine.
4. Season with salt and pepper and serve.

Nutritional Information: calories: 330; carbohydrates: 40g; protein: 16g; fat: 14g; fiber: 10g; vitamins: A, C; potassium: 600mg; sodium: 300mg; sugar: 3g.

Zucchini Noodles with Pesto and Grilled Chicken

Preparation Time: 10 minutes   **Cooking Time:** 15 minutes   **Servings:** 2

INGREDIENTS:

- 2 zucchinis, spiralized
- 1/2 cup pesto sauce (dairy-free if needed)
- 2 chicken breasts
- 1 tbsp olive oil
- Salt and pepper to taste

PREPARATION:

1. Grill chicken breasts for 6-7 minutes on each side or until fully cooked. Slice and set aside.
2. In a large bowl, toss spiralized zucchini with pesto sauce.
3. Serve zucchini noodles topped with grilled chicken slices.
4. Season with salt and pepper.

Nutritional Information: calories: 380; carbohydrates: 12g; protein: 36g; fat: 22g; fiber: 4g; vitamins: A, C; potassium: 800mg; sodium: 400mg; sugar: 4g.

Grilled Chicken Salad with Walnuts and Balsamic Vinaigrette

Preparation Time: 10 minutes   **Cooking Time:** 15 minutes   **Servings:** 2

INGREDIENTS:

- 2 chicken breasts
- 4 cups mixed greens
- 1/4 cup walnuts, chopped
- 1/4 cup balsamic vinaigrette
- 1 tbsp olive oil
- Salt and pepper to taste

PREPARATION:

1. Grill chicken breasts for 6-7 minutes on each side or until fully cooked. Slice and set aside.
2. In a bowl, combine mixed greens and walnuts.
3. Drizzle with balsamic vinaigrette and toss gently.
4. Serve with grilled chicken slices on top.

Nutritional Information: calories: 410; carbohydrates: 14g; protein: 36g; fat: 25g; fiber: 6g; vitamins: A, C, K; potassium: 700mg; sodium: 200mg; sugar: 6g.

Tofu Stir-Fry with Broccoli and Brown Rice

Preparation Time: 10 minutes   **Cooking Time:** 15 minutes   **Servings:** 2

INGREDIENTS:

- 200g firm tofu, cubed
- 1 cup broccoli florets
- 1/2 cup cooked brown rice
- 2 tbsp soy sauce (gluten-free if needed)
- 1 tbsp olive oil
- 1 tsp sesame seeds

PREPARATION:

1. Heat olive oil in a pan over medium heat. Add tofu and cook until golden brown, about 5 minutes. Remove and set aside.
2. In the same pan, sauté broccoli until tender, about 3-4 minutes.
3. Stir in cooked brown rice and tofu. Drizzle with soy sauce and sprinkle with sesame seeds.
4. Serve immediately.

Nutritional Information: calories: 350; carbohydrates: 42g; protein: 15g; fat: 15g; fiber: 6g; vitamins: A, C, K; potassium: 400mg; sodium: 500mg; sugar: 4g.

Wild Rice Salad with Roasted Vegetables and Almonds

Preparation Time: 10 minutes   **Cooking Time:** 25 minutes   **Servings:** 2

INGREDIENTS:

- 1/2 cup wild rice
- 1 cup roasted vegetables (e.g., bell peppers, zucchini)
- 1/4 cup almonds, chopped
- 2 tbsp olive oil
- 1 tbsp balsamic vinegar
- Salt and pepper to taste

PREPARATION:

1. Cook wild rice according to package instructions. Let cool.
2. In a large bowl, combine wild rice, roasted vegetables, and almonds.
3. Drizzle with olive oil and balsamic vinegar, then toss to combine.
4. Season with salt and pepper and serve.

Nutritional Information: calories: 320; carbohydrates: 45g; protein: 9g; fat: 12g; fiber: 7g; vitamins: A, C; potassium: 500mg; sodium: 300mg; sugar: 5g.

Tuna Salad with Mixed Greens and Lemon Olive Oil Dressing

Preparation Time: 10 minutes   **Cooking Time:** 0 minutes   **Servings:** 2

INGREDIENTS:

- 1 can tuna in water, drained
- 4 cups mixed greens
- 1/2 avocado, sliced
- 1/2 cup cherry tomatoes, halved
- 2 tbsp olive oil
- 1 tbsp lemon juice
- Salt and pepper to taste

PREPARATION:

1. In a large bowl, combine mixed greens, tuna, avocado, and cherry tomatoes.
2. Drizzle with olive oil and lemon juice. Toss gently.
3. Season with salt and pepper and serve.

Nutritional Information: calories: 350; carbohydrates: 12g; protein: 30g; fat: 22g; fiber: 6g; vitamins: A, C, K; potassium: 800mg; sodium: 300mg; sugar: 4g.

Chickpea and Quinoa Buddha Bowl with Tahini Dressing

Preparation Time: 15 minutes   **Cooking Time:** 20 minutes   **Servings:** 2

INGREDIENTS:

- 1/2 cup quinoa, rinsed
- 1/2 cup canned chickpeas, drained and rinsed
- 1/4 cup shredded carrots
- 1/2 avocado, sliced
- 1/4 cucumber, sliced
- 1/4 cup cherry tomatoes, halved
- 2 tbsp tahini
- 1 tbsp lemon juice
- 1 tbsp water
- Salt and pepper to taste

PREPARATION:

1. Cook quinoa according to package instructions. Let it cool.
2. In a bowl, layer quinoa, chickpeas, carrots, avocado, cucumber, and cherry tomatoes.
3. In a small bowl, mix tahini, lemon juice, water, salt, and pepper to make the dressing.
4. Drizzle dressing over the Buddha bowl and serve.

Nutritional Information: calories: 400; carbohydrates: 50g; protein: 14g; fat: 18g; fiber: 12g; vitamins: A, C, K; potassium: 700mg; sodium: 250mg; sugar: 4g.

Spinach and Mushroom Frittata

Preparation Time: 10 minutes   **Cooking Time:** 20 minutes   **Servings:** 2

INGREDIENTS:

- 4 large eggs
- 1/2 cup fresh spinach, chopped
- 1/4 cup mushrooms, sliced
- 1/4 cup feta cheese (omit for dairy-free)
- 1 tbsp olive oil
- Salt and pepper to taste

PREPARATION:

1. Preheat the oven to 350°F (175°C).
2. Heat olive oil in an oven-safe skillet over medium heat. Add mushrooms and spinach, cooking until tender.
3. In a bowl, whisk eggs, salt, and pepper. Pour the mixture over the veggies in the skillet.
4. Add feta cheese on top and transfer the skillet to the oven. Bake for 15 minutes or until the eggs are set.

Nutritional Information: calories: 320; carbohydrates: 5g; protein: 22g; fat: 24g; fiber: 2g; vitamins: A, D, K; potassium: 350mg; sodium: 450mg; sugar: 1g.

Salmon and Avocado Sushi Bowl

Preparation Time: 15 minutes   **Cooking Time:** 20 minutes   **Servings:** 2

INGREDIENTS:

- 1/2 cup sushi rice
- 2 salmon fillets, grilled
- 1 avocado, sliced
- 1/2 cucumber, sliced
- 1 tbsp soy sauce (gluten-free if needed)
- 1 tbsp rice vinegar
- 1 tsp sesame seeds

PREPARATION:

1. Cook sushi rice according to package instructions, then mix in rice vinegar.
2. In a bowl, layer the sushi rice, grilled salmon, avocado, and cucumber.
3. Drizzle with soy sauce and sprinkle sesame seeds on top.
4. Serve immediately.

Nutritional Information: calories: 450; carbohydrates: 45g; protein: 28g; fat: 18g; fiber: 6g; vitamins: A, C; potassium: 900mg; sodium: 400mg; sugar: 3g.

Roasted Sweet Potato and Lentil Salad

Preparation Time: 15 minutes **Cooking Time:** 25 minutes **Servings:** 2

INGREDIENTS:

- 1 sweet potato, diced
- 1/2 cup green lentils
- 2 tbsp olive oil
- 1/4 cup red onion, sliced
- 1/4 cup parsley, chopped
- Salt and pepper to taste

PREPARATION:

1. Preheat oven to 400°F (200°C). Toss sweet potato in olive oil, salt, and pepper, and roast for 20 minutes until tender.
2. Cook lentils according to package instructions. Drain and cool.
3. In a bowl, combine roasted sweet potato, lentils, red onion, and parsley.
4. Drizzle with remaining olive oil, toss, and serve.

Nutritional Information: calories: 380; carbohydrates: 55g; protein: 14g; fat: 10g; fiber: 14g; vitamins: A, C, K; potassium: 900mg; sodium: 200mg; sugar: 8g.

Grilled Shrimp with Quinoa and Arugula Salad

Preparation Time: 10 minutes **Cooking Time:** 15 minutes **Servings:** 2

INGREDIENTS:

- 1/2 cup quinoa, rinsed
- 12 large shrimp, peeled and deveined
- 2 cups arugula
- 1/4 cup cherry tomatoes, halved
- 1 tbsp olive oil
- 1 tbsp lemon juice
- Salt and pepper to taste

PREPARATION:

1. Cook quinoa according to package instructions and let cool.
2. Grill shrimp for 2-3 minutes on each side until cooked.
3. In a bowl, combine arugula, cherry tomatoes, and quinoa.
4. Drizzle with olive oil and lemon juice, then toss gently.
5. Serve topped with grilled shrimp.

Nutritional Information: calories: 400; carbohydrates: 34g; protein: 26g; fat: 15g; fiber: 5g; vitamins: A, C, K; potassium: 800mg; sodium: 350mg; sugar: 3g.

CHAPTER 6

Dinner Recipes

Baked Lemon Herb Salmon with Quinoa and Steamed Asparagus

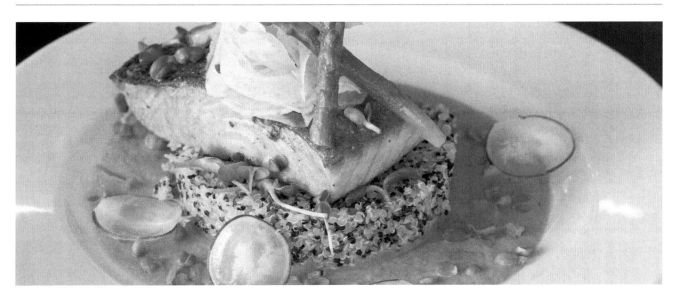

Preparation Time: 10 minutes   **Cooking Time:** 25 minutes   **Servings:** 2

INGREDIENTS:

- 2 salmon fillets
- 1/2 cup quinoa
- 1 bunch asparagus, trimmed
- 1 tbsp olive oil
- Juice of 1 lemon
- 1 tbsp fresh parsley, chopped
- 1 tsp dried thyme
- Salt and pepper to taste

PREPARATION:

1. Preheat the oven to 375°F (190°C).
2. Place the salmon fillets on a baking sheet and drizzle with olive oil, lemon juice, parsley, thyme, salt, and pepper. Bake for 20 minutes or until cooked through.
3. Cook quinoa according to package instructions.
4. Steam the asparagus for 5 minutes or until tender.
5. Serve the baked salmon with quinoa and steamed asparagus.

Nutritional Information: calories: 420; carbohydrates: 35g; protein: 38g; fat: 16g; fiber: 5g; vitamins: C, D; potassium: 900mg; sodium: 160mg; sugar: 2g.

Chicken and Sweet Potato Curry with Brown Rice

Preparation Time: 15 minutes   **Cooking Time:** 30 minutes   **Servings:** 4

INGREDIENTS:

- 2 chicken breasts, diced
- 1 large sweet potato, diced
- 1 cup brown rice
- 1 can coconut milk
- 2 tbsp curry powder
- 1 onion, diced
- 1 tbsp olive oil
- 1 tsp ground cumin
- Salt and pepper to taste

PREPARATION:

1. Cook brown rice according to package instructions.
2. In a large pan, heat olive oil and sauté the onion until soft.
3. Add chicken and cook until browned.
4. Add sweet potato, coconut milk, curry powder, cumin, salt, and pepper. Simmer for 20 minutes or until the sweet potato is tender.
5. Serve the curry over brown rice.

Nutritional Information: calories: 450; carbohydrates: 48g; protein: 30g; fat: 15g; fiber: 6g; vitamins: A, C; potassium: 780mg; sodium: 300mg; sugar: 5g.

Grilled Tofu Steaks with Sautéed Spinach and Quinoa

Preparation Time: 10 minutes   **Cooking Time:** 20 minutes   **Servings:** 2

INGREDIENTS:

- 1 block firm tofu, sliced into steaks
- 1 tbsp olive oil
- 1/2 cup quinoa
- 4 cups spinach
- 1 clove garlic, minced
- 1 tbsp soy sauce or tamari (for gluten-free)
- Salt and pepper to taste

PREPARATION:

1. Cook quinoa according to package instructions.
2. Heat olive oil in a grill pan and cook tofu steaks for 4-5 minutes on each side.
3. In a separate pan, sauté garlic and spinach until wilted.
4. Serve the tofu steaks with sautéed spinach and quinoa. Drizzle with soy sauce or tamari.

Nutritional Information: calories: 350; carbohydrates: 35g; protein: 24g; fat: 16g; fiber: 5g; vitamins: C, A; potassium: 850mg; sodium: 400mg; sugar: 2g.

Seared Tuna with Spinach and Brown Rice

Preparation Time: 10 minutes   **Cooking Time:** 20 minutes   **Servings:** 2

INGREDIENTS:

- 2 tuna steaks
- 2 cups spinach
- 1 cup cooked brown rice
- 1 tbsp olive oil
- 1 tbsp soy sauce or tamari
- Juice of 1 lime
- 1 clove garlic, minced
- Salt and pepper to taste

PREPARATION:

1. Heat olive oil in a pan over medium–high heat. Season tuna steaks with salt and pepper, and sear for 2–3 minutes per side for medium-rare. Remove from the pan.
2. In the same pan, sauté garlic and spinach for 2 minutes until wilted.
3. Serve seared tuna over brown rice, with spinach on the side, and drizzle with lime juice and soy sauce.

Nutritional Information: calories: 420; carbohydrates: 30g; protein: 40g; fat: 15g; fiber: 5g; vitamins: A, C; potassium: 700mg; sodium: 600mg; sugar: 3g.

Turkey Meatballs with Zucchini Noodles and Marinara Sauce

Preparation Time: 15 minutes   **Cooking Time:** 25 minutes   **Servings:** 4

INGREDIENTS:

- 1 lb ground turkey
- 1 egg
- 1/4 cup almond flour
- 1 tbsp fresh parsley, chopped
- Salt and pepper to taste
- 2 large zucchinis, spiralized
- 1 cup marinara sauce

PREPARATION:

1. Preheat the oven to 375°F (190°C).
2. In a bowl, mix ground turkey, egg, almond flour, parsley, salt, and pepper. Form into meatballs.
3. Place the meatballs on a baking sheet and bake for 20 minutes.
4. Meanwhile, heat the marinara sauce in a pan and lightly sauté the zucchini noodles.
5. Serve meatballs over zucchini noodles and top with marinara sauce.

Nutritional Information: calories: 320; carbohydrates: 12g; protein: 35g; fat: 14g; fiber: 3g; vitamins: A, C; potassium: 740mg; sodium: 450mg; sugar: 4g.

Grilled Mahi-Mahi with Mango Salsa and Brown Rice

Preparation Time: 10 minutes   **Cooking Time:** 20 minutes   **Servings:** 2

INGREDIENTS:

- 2 mahi-mahi fillets
- 1 cup brown rice
- 1/2 mango, diced
- 1/4 cup red onion, finely chopped
- 1 tbsp fresh cilantro, chopped
- Juice of 1 lime
- 1 tbsp olive oil
- Salt and pepper to taste

PREPARATION:

1. Cook brown rice according to package instructions.
2. Grill mahi-mahi fillets for 5-6 minutes per side, brushing with olive oil.
3. In a bowl, mix diced mango, red onion, cilantro, lime juice, salt, and pepper to make the salsa.
4. Serve grilled mahi-mahi with brown rice and mango salsa on top.

Nutritional Information: calories: 400; carbohydrates: 45g; protein: 30g; fat: 10g; fiber: 6g; vitamins: C, D; potassium: 700mg; sodium: 120mg; sugar: 10g.

Lentil and Vegetable Stew with Fresh Herbs

Preparation Time: 10 minutes   **Cooking Time:** 30 minutes   **Servings:** 4

INGREDIENTS:

- 1 cup dried lentils, rinsed
- 1 carrot, diced
- 1 zucchini, diced
- 1 onion, chopped
- 2 cloves garlic, minced
- 1 can diced tomatoes
- 4 cups vegetable broth
- 1 tbsp olive oil
- 1 tbsp fresh thyme
- Salt and pepper to taste

PREPARATION:

1. Heat olive oil in a large pot and sauté onions, garlic, and carrots for 5 minutes.
2. Add lentils, diced tomatoes, zucchini, vegetable broth, thyme, salt, and pepper. Bring to a boil.
3. Reduce heat and simmer for 25 minutes, stirring occasionally, until lentils are tender.
4. Garnish with fresh herbs and serve hot.

Nutritional Information: calories: 280; carbohydrates: 40g; protein: 14g; fat: 7g; fiber: 15g; vitamins: A, C; potassium: 700mg; sodium: 450mg; sugar: 8g.

Baked Chicken Breast with Roasted Brussels Sprouts and Sweet Potatoes

Preparation Time: 15 minutes   **Cooking Time:** 30 minutes   **Servings:** 4

INGREDIENTS:

- 4 boneless, skinless chicken breasts
- 2 cups Brussels sprouts, halved
- 2 medium sweet potatoes, diced
- 2 tbsp olive oil
- 1 tbsp fresh rosemary, chopped
- Salt and pepper to taste

PREPARATION:

1. Preheat oven to 400°F (200°C).
2. Toss Brussels sprouts and sweet potatoes with 1 tbsp olive oil, rosemary, salt, and pepper. Spread on a baking sheet.
3. Rub chicken breasts with remaining olive oil, salt, and pepper. Place on another baking sheet.
4. Roast vegetables and chicken for 25-30 minutes, until chicken is fully cooked and vegetables are tender.
5. Serve chicken with roasted vegetables.

Nutritional Information: calories: 450; carbohydrates: 35g; protein: 42g; fat: 18g; fiber: 7g; vitamins: A, C; potassium: 900mg; sodium: 350mg; sugar: 6g.

Grilled Cod with Olive Oil, Lemon, and Asparagus

Preparation Time: 10 minutes   **Cooking Time:** 15 minutes   **Servings:** 2

INGREDIENTS:

- 2 cod fillets
- 1 bunch asparagus, trimmed
- 2 tbsp olive oil
- Juice of 1 lemon
- 1 tsp lemon zest
- Salt and pepper to taste

PREPARATION:

1. Preheat grill to medium-high heat.
2. Drizzle cod fillets with 1 tbsp olive oil, lemon juice, lemon zest, salt, and pepper. Grill for 5-6 minutes per side.
3. Toss asparagus with remaining olive oil, salt, and pepper. Grill for 5 minutes, turning occasionally.
4. Serve grilled cod with asparagus.

Nutritional Information: calories: 310; carbohydrates: 8g; protein: 30g; fat: 18g; fiber: 4g; vitamins: C, D; potassium: 700mg; sodium: 150mg; sugar: 3g.

Black Bean and Quinoa Stuffed Peppers

Preparation Time: 15 minutes   **Cooking Time:** 25 minutes   **Servings:** 4

INGREDIENTS:

- 4 large bell peppers, halved and seeds removed
- 1 cup cooked quinoa
- 1 can black beans, drained and rinsed
- 1/2 cup corn kernels
- 1/4 cup salsa
- 1 tsp cumin
- Salt and pepper to taste
- 1 tbsp olive oil

PREPARATION:

1. Preheat oven to 375°F (190°C).
2. In a large bowl, combine quinoa, black beans, corn, salsa, cumin, salt, and pepper.
3. Stuff the bell pepper halves with the quinoa mixture.
4. Place stuffed peppers on a baking sheet, drizzle with olive oil, and bake for 25 minutes.
5. Serve warm.

Nutritional Information: calories: 260; carbohydrates: 40g; protein: 10g; fat: 8g; fiber: 8g; vitamins: C, A; potassium: 600mg; sodium: 300mg; sugar: 7g.

Sautéed Shrimp with Broccoli and Brown Rice

Preparation Time: 10 minutes   **Cooking Time:** 20 minutes   **Servings:** 2

INGREDIENTS:

- 1/2 lb shrimp, peeled and deveined
- 2 cups broccoli florets
- 1 cup cooked brown rice
- 1 tbsp olive oil
- 1 clove garlic, minced
- 1 tbsp soy sauce or tamari
- 1/2 tsp ginger, grated
- Salt and pepper to taste

PREPARATION:

1. Heat olive oil in a large pan over medium heat. Add garlic and ginger, and sauté for 1 minute.
2. Add shrimp to the pan and cook for 3-4 minutes until pink. Remove and set aside.
3. Add broccoli to the pan, cover, and cook for 5 minutes, until tender.
4. Return shrimp to the pan and drizzle with soy sauce or tamari.
5. Serve with cooked brown rice.

Nutritional Information: calories: 350; carbohydrates: 42g; protein: 28g; fat: 10g; fiber: 5g; vitamins: C, D; potassium: 650mg; sodium: 400mg; sugar: 2g.

Baked Cod with Wild Rice and Green Beans

Preparation Time: 10 minutes   **Cooking Time:** 25 minutes   **Servings:** 2

INGREDIENTS:

- 2 cod fillets
- 1 cup wild rice
- 1/2 lb green beans, trimmed
- 1 tbsp olive oil
- Juice of 1 lemon
- Salt and pepper to taste

PREPARATION:

1. Cook wild rice according to package instructions.
2. Preheat oven to 375°F (190°C).
3. Place cod fillets on a baking sheet, drizzle with olive oil, lemon juice, salt, and pepper. Bake for 20 minutes or until cooked through.
4. Steam green beans for 5 minutes or until tender.
5. Serve baked cod with wild rice and steamed green beans.

Nutritional Information: calories: 390; carbohydrates: 45g; protein: 30g; fat: 12g; fiber: 7g; vitamins: C, D; potassium: 750mg; sodium: 180mg; sugar: 4g.

Roasted Vegetable and Chickpea Tagine

Preparation Time: 15 minutes   **Cooking Time:** 35 minutes   **Servings:** 4

INGREDIENTS:

- 1 can chickpeas, drained and rinsed
- 1 large carrot, diced
- 1 zucchini, diced
- 1 red bell pepper, chopped
- 1 onion, chopped
- 2 cloves garlic, minced
- 1 can diced tomatoes
- 1/2 tsp ground cumin
- 1/2 tsp ground coriander
- 1/2 tsp ground cinnamon
- 1/4 tsp turmeric
- 1 tbsp olive oil
- Salt and pepper to taste
- 1/4 cup fresh cilantro, chopped (optional)

PREPARATION:

1. Preheat the oven to 375°F (190°C).
2. Toss the carrots, zucchini, bell pepper, and onion with olive oil, salt, and pepper. Spread on a baking sheet and roast for 20-25 minutes until vegetables are tender.
3. In a large pot, heat olive oil and sauté garlic for 1 minute. Add diced tomatoes, chickpeas, cumin, coriander, cinnamon, and turmeric. Simmer for 10 minutes.
4. Add roasted vegetables to the pot and stir well. Simmer for an additional 5 minutes.
5. Serve with chopped cilantro on top, if desired.

Nutritional Information: calories: 320; carbohydrates: 50g; protein: 12g; fat: 10g; fiber: 10g; vitamins: A, C; potassium: 780mg; sodium: 430mg; sugar: 10g.

Grilled Portobello Mushrooms with Quinoa and Sautéed Kale

Preparation Time: 10 minutes   **Cooking Time:** 20 minutes   **Servings:** 2

INGREDIENTS:

- 2 large Portobello mushrooms
- 1 cup cooked quinoa
- 2 cups kale, chopped
- 1 clove garlic, minced
- 1 tbsp olive oil
- 1 tsp balsamic vinegar
- Salt and pepper to taste

PREPARATION:

1. Preheat grill to medium-high heat. Brush Portobello mushrooms with olive oil, salt, and pepper, and grill for 5-7 minutes per side.
2. In a pan, heat olive oil and sauté garlic and kale for 3-4 minutes until kale wilts. Add balsamic vinegar and season with salt and pepper.
3. Serve grilled mushrooms on a bed of quinoa with sautéed kale on the side.

Nutritional Information: calories: 290; carbohydrates: 42g; protein: 12g; fat: 9g; fiber: 7g; vitamins: A, C, K; potassium: 620mg; sodium: 270mg; sugar: 4g.

Turkey Chili with Kidney Beans and Avocado

Preparation Time: 10 minutes   **Cooking Time:** 30 minutes   **Servings:** 4

INGREDIENTS:

- 1 lb ground turkey
- 1 can kidney beans, drained and rinsed
- 1 can diced tomatoes
- 1 small onion, chopped
- 1 clove garlic, minced
- 1 tbsp olive oil
- 1 tbsp chili powder
- 1 tsp cumin
- Salt and pepper to taste
- 1 avocado, sliced

PREPARATION:

1. Heat olive oil in a large pot over medium heat. Add onion and garlic, and sauté for 3-4 minutes until softened.
2. Add ground turkey, chili powder, cumin, salt, and pepper. Cook until the turkey is browned, about 5-6 minutes.
3. Add kidney beans and diced tomatoes, reduce heat, and simmer for 20 minutes.
4. Serve turkey chili topped with avocado slices.

Nutritional Information: calories: 380; carbohydrates: 24g; protein: 35g; fat: 17g; fiber: 10g; vitamins: A, C; potassium: 890mg; sodium: 450mg; sugar: 5g.

CHAPTER 7

Dessert Recipes

Coconut Chia Seed Pudding with Mango

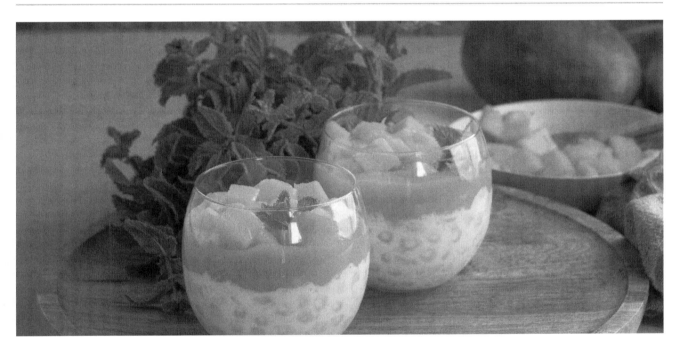

Preparation Time: 10 minutes

Cooking Time: 0 minutes
(plus 4 hours refrigeration)

Servings: 2

INGREDIENTS:

- 1/4 cup chia seeds
- 1 cup coconut milk
- 1 tbsp maple syrup (optional)
- 1/2 mango, diced

PREPARATION:

1. In a bowl, combine chia seeds, coconut milk, and maple syrup. Stir well.
2. Let the mixture sit for 5 minutes, then stir again to break up any clumps.
3. Refrigerate for at least 4 hours or overnight until the pudding is set.
4. Top with diced mango before serving.

Nutritional Information: calories: 250; carbohydrates: 32g; protein: 5g; fat: 12g; fiber: 10g; vitamins: A, C; potassium: 300mg; sodium: 45mg; sugar: 15g.

Dark Chocolate Almond Bark

Preparation Time: 10 minutes   **Cooking Time:** 10 minutes   **Servings:** 4

INGREDIENTS:

- 1 cup dark chocolate (70% cocoa or higher)
- 1/4 cup almonds, chopped
- 1 tbsp coconut flakes

PREPARATION:

1. Melt the dark chocolate in a double boiler or microwave, stirring frequently.
2. Spread melted chocolate onto a parchment-lined baking sheet in a thin layer.
3. Sprinkle chopped almonds and coconut flakes evenly over the chocolate.
4. Refrigerate for about 30 minutes or until fully set.
5. Break into pieces and serve.

Nutritional Information: calories: 220; carbohydrates: 20g; protein: 4g; fat: 15g; fiber: 5g; vitamins: E; potassium: 200mg; sodium: 10mg; sugar: 12g.

Pumpkin Spice Smoothie Bowl

Preparation Time: 5 minutes   **Cooking Time:** 0 minutes   **Servings:** 2

INGREDIENTS:

- 1/2 cup pumpkin puree
- 1/2 banana
- 1/2 tsp cinnamon
- 1/4 tsp nutmeg
- 1/4 cup almond milk
- 1 tbsp chia seeds

PREPARATION:

1. In a blender, combine pumpkin puree, banana, cinnamon, nutmeg, almond milk, and chia seeds. Blend until smooth.
2. Pour into bowls and top with your favorite toppings, such as granola or chopped nuts.

Nutritional Information: calories: 160; carbohydrates: 30g; protein: 4g; fat: 5g; fiber: 7g; vitamins: A, C; potassium: 300mg; sodium: 30mg; sugar: 10g.

Baked Apples with Cinnamon and Walnuts

Preparation Time: 10 minutes   **Cooking Time:** 25 minutes   **Servings:** 2

INGREDIENTS:

- 2 apples, cored
- 2 tbsp walnuts, chopped
- 1 tsp cinnamon
- 1 tbsp maple syrup (optional)

PREPARATION:

1. Preheat oven to 350°F (175°C).
2. Place the cored apples in a baking dish.
3. In a small bowl, mix walnuts, cinnamon, and maple syrup. Stuff the mixture into the apples.
4. Bake for 25 minutes or until apples are tender.

Nutritional Information: calories: 200; carbohydrates: 40g; protein: 2g; fat: 5g; fiber: 7g; vitamins: C; potassium: 250mg; sodium: 5mg; sugar: 25g.

Greek Yogurt with Honey and Pistachios

Preparation Time: 5 minutes   **Cooking Time:** 0 minutes   **Servings:** 2

INGREDIENTS:

- 1 cup Greek yogurt
- 1 tbsp honey
- 2 tbsp pistachios, chopped

PREPARATION:

1. Divide Greek yogurt into two bowls.
2. Drizzle honey on top of each serving.
3. Sprinkle with chopped pistachios and serve.

Nutritional Information: calories: 200; carbohydrates: 18g; protein: 10g; fat: 8g; fiber: 2g; vitamins: D; potassium: 250mg; sodium: 60mg; sugar: 15g.

Almond Butter and Dark Chocolate Energy Bites

Preparation Time: 10 minutes   **Cooking Time:** 0 minutes   **Servings:** 6

INGREDIENTS:

- 1/2 cup almond butter
- 1/4 cup dark chocolate chips
- 1/4 cup oats
- 1 tbsp chia seeds
- 1 tbsp honey (optional)

PREPARATION:

1. In a bowl, combine almond butter, oats, chia seeds, and honey (if using). Stir well.
2. Fold in dark chocolate chips.
3. Roll the mixture into small balls and place on a baking sheet.
4. Refrigerate for at least 30 minutes before serving.

Nutritional Information: calories: 180; carbohydrates: 15g; protein: 6g; fat: 12g; fiber: 4g; vitamins: E; potassium: 180mg; sodium: 40mg; sugar: 8g.

Berry and Almond Parfait

Preparation Time: 5 minutes   **Cooking Time:** 0 minutes   **Servings:** 2

INGREDIENTS:

- 1/2 cup mixed berries
- 1/2 cup Greek yogurt (or coconut yogurt for dairy-free)
- 1 tbsp almond butter
- 1 tbsp almonds, chopped

PREPARATION:

1. In serving glasses, layer Greek yogurt, mixed berries, and almond butter.
2. Top with chopped almonds.
3. Serve immediately.

Nutritional Information: calories: 180; carbohydrates: 20g; protein: 7g; fat: 10g; fiber: 4g; vitamins: A, C, E; potassium: 250mg; sodium: 40mg; sugar: 12g.

Avocado Chocolate Mousse

Preparation Time: 10 minutes   **Cooking Time:** 0 minutes   **Servings:** 2

INGREDIENTS:

- 1 ripe avocado
- 1/4 cup cocoa powder
- 2 tbsp maple syrup
- 1/4 cup almond milk

PREPARATION:

1. In a blender, combine avocado, cocoa powder, maple syrup, and almond milk. Blend until smooth.
2. Divide into serving dishes and refrigerate for 30 minutes before serving.

Nutritional Information: calories: 220; carbohydrates: 25g; protein: 3g; fat: 15g; fiber: 7g; vitamins: C; potassium: 500mg; sodium: 20mg; sugar: 15g.

Banana Ice Cream with Almond Butter Swirl

Preparation Time: 10 minutes   **Cooking Time:** 0 minutes   **Servings:** 2

INGREDIENTS:

- 2 frozen bananas
- 1 tbsp almond butter
- 1/2 tsp vanilla extract

PREPARATION:

1. Blend frozen bananas and vanilla extract in a blender until creamy.
2. Swirl in almond butter and mix gently.
3. Serve immediately or freeze for a firmer texture.

Nutritional Information: calories: 180; carbohydrates: 35g; protein: 2g; fat: 4g; fiber: 4g; vitamins: C; potassium: 500mg; sodium: 0mg; sugar: 20g.

Warm Pear and Walnut Crumble

Preparation Time: 10 minutes   **Cooking Time:** 25 minutes   **Servings:** 2

INGREDIENTS:

- 2 pears, sliced
- 1/4 cup walnuts, chopped
- 1 tbsp coconut oil
- 1 tbsp maple syrup
- 1/4 cup oats (gluten-free)
- 1/2 tsp cinnamon

PREPARATION:

1. Preheat oven to 350°F (175°C).
2. In a small bowl, mix the oats, walnuts, coconut oil, and maple syrup.
3. Place sliced pears in a baking dish and top with the oat mixture.
4. Sprinkle with cinnamon.
5. Bake for 25 minutes or until the topping is golden brown.

Nutritional Information: calories: 250; carbohydrates: 40g; protein: 4g; fat: 10g; fiber: 6g; vitamins: C; potassium: 300mg; sodium: 5mg; sugar: 20g.

Lemon Chia Seed Pudding

Preparation Time: 10 minutes   **Cooking Time:** 0 minutes (plus 4 hours refrigeration)   **Servings:** 2

INGREDIENTS:

- 1/4 cup chia seeds
- 1 cup almond milk
- 1 tbsp lemon juice
- 1 tbsp maple syrup
- 1 tsp lemon zest

PREPARATION:

1. In a bowl, combine chia seeds, almond milk, lemon juice, maple syrup, and lemon zest. Stir well.
2. Let the mixture sit for 5 minutes, then stir again to break up any clumps.
3. Refrigerate for at least 4 hours or overnight until set.
4. Serve chilled and garnish with extra lemon zest if desired.

Nutritional Information: calories: 220; carbohydrates: 25g; protein: 5g; fat: 11g; fiber: 8g; vitamins: C; potassium: 180mg; sodium: 50mg; sugar: 12g.

Blueberry and Oatmeal Bars

Preparation Time: 15 minutes   **Cooking Time:** 25 minutes   **Servings:** 6

INGREDIENTS:

- 1 1/2 cups rolled oats (gluten-free)
- 1/2 cup almond flour
- 1/4 cup coconut oil, melted
- 1/4 cup maple syrup
- 1 tsp vanilla extract
- 1 cup fresh blueberries

PREPARATION:

1. Preheat oven to 350°F (175°C). Line a baking pan with parchment paper.
2. In a large bowl, mix oats, almond flour, coconut oil, maple syrup, and vanilla.
3. Press half the mixture into the pan.
4. Spread blueberries over the oat mixture.
5. Crumble the remaining oat mixture on top.
6. Bake for 25 minutes or until golden brown.
7. Let cool before cutting into bars.

Nutritional Information: calories: 240; carbohydrates: 30g; protein: 5g; fat: 12g; fiber: 5g; vitamins: A, C; potassium: 120mg; sodium: 50mg; sugar: 14g.

Dark Chocolate-Covered Strawberries

Preparation Time: 10 minutes   **Cooking Time:** 10 minutes   **Servings:** 2

INGREDIENTS:

- 1/2 cup dark chocolate chips (70% cocoa or higher)
- 1 cup fresh strawberries

PREPARATION:

1. Melt dark chocolate in a double boiler or microwave, stirring frequently.
2. Dip strawberries into the melted chocolate and place on parchment paper.
3. Refrigerate for 30 minutes or until the chocolate is set.
4. Serve chilled.

Nutritional Information: calories: 180; carbohydrates: 25g; protein: 2g; fat: 8g; fiber: 4g; vitamins: C; potassium: 200mg; sodium: 10mg; sugar: 15g.

Roasted Peach with Honey and Almonds

Preparation Time: 5 minutes   **Cooking Time:** 15 minutes   **Servings:** 2

INGREDIENTS:

- 2 ripe peaches, halved
- 1 tbsp honey
- 2 tbsp sliced almonds
- 1/2 tsp cinnamon

PREPARATION:

1. Preheat oven to 375°F (190°C).
2. Place peach halves on a baking sheet.
3. Drizzle honey over the peaches and sprinkle with cinnamon.
4. Roast for 15 minutes until tender.
5. Top with sliced almonds and serve.

Nutritional Information: calories: 180; carbohydrates: 30g; protein: 3g; fat: 5g; fiber: 4g; vitamins: C; potassium: 250mg; sodium: 5mg; sugar: 22g.

Raspberry and Coconut Energy Balls

Preparation Time: 10 minutes   **Cooking Time:** 0 minutes   **Servings:** 6

INGREDIENTS:

- 1/2 cup shredded coconut
- 1/2 cup oats (gluten-free)
- 1/4 cup dried raspberries
- 2 tbsp almond butter
- 1 tbsp honey

PREPARATION:

1. In a food processor, blend all ingredients until well combined.
2. Roll the mixture into small balls and place on a baking sheet.
3. Refrigerate for at least 30 minutes before serving.

Nutritional Information: calories: 150; carbohydrates: 20g; protein: 3g; fat: 7g; fiber: 3g; vitamins: C; potassium: 150mg; sodium: 30mg; sugar: 12g.

CHAPTER 8

Snack Recipes

Almonds and Dried Cranberries Trail Mix

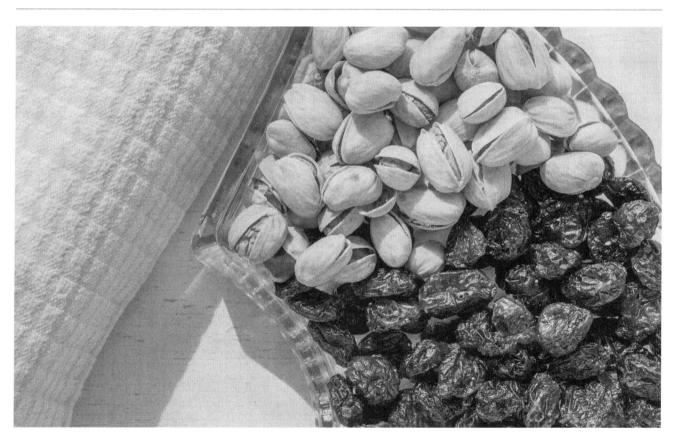

Preparation Time: 5 minutes   **Cooking Time:** 0 minutes   **Servings:** 2

INGREDIENTS:

- 1/4 cup raw almonds
- 1/4 cup dried cranberries (no added sugar)
- 2 tbsp pumpkin seeds

PREPARATION:

1. In a small bowl, mix almonds, dried cranberries, and pumpkin seeds.
2. Serve as a quick snack or pack for on-the-go.

Nutritional Information: calories: 200; carbohydrates: 22g; protein: 5g; fat: 10g; fiber: 5g; vitamins: E; potassium: 220mg; sodium: 10mg; sugar: 13g.

Roasted Chickpeas with
Sea Salt and Paprika

Preparation Time: 5 minutes **Cooking Time:** 30 minutes **Servings:** 2

INGREDIENTS:

- 1 cup cooked chickpeas
- 1 tbsp olive oil
- 1/2 tsp sea salt
- 1/2 tsp paprika

PREPARATION:

1. Preheat oven to 400°F (200°C).
2. Toss chickpeas with olive oil, sea salt, and paprika.
3. Spread chickpeas on a baking sheet and roast for 30 minutes, shaking halfway through.
4. Let cool slightly before serving.

Nutritional Information: calories: 180; carbohydrates: 25g; protein: 6g; fat: 6g; fiber: 7g; vitamins: A; potassium: 240mg; sodium: 300mg; sugar: 2g.

Veggie Sticks with Hummus

Preparation Time: 10 minutes **Cooking Time:** 0 minutes **Servings:** 2

INGREDIENTS:

- 1 carrot, sliced
- 1 cucumber, sliced
- 1/4 cup hummus

PREPARATION:

1. Arrange veggie sticks on a plate.
2. Serve with hummus for dipping.

Nutritional Information: calories: 120; carbohydrates: 18g; protein: 3g; fat: 5g; fiber: 5g; vitamins: A, C; potassium: 300mg; sodium: 120mg; sugar: 4g.

Sliced Apple with Almond Butter and Cinnamon

Preparation Time: 5 minutes   **Cooking Time:** 0 minutes   **Servings:** 1

INGREDIENTS:

- 1 medium apple, sliced
- 1 tbsp almond butter
- 1/4 tsp cinnamon

PREPARATION:

1. Arrange apple slices on a plate.
2. Spread almond butter on each slice.
3. Sprinkle with cinnamon and enjoy.

Nutritional Information: calories: 180; carbohydrates: 25g; protein: 4g; fat: 8g; fiber: 5g; vitamins: C; potassium: 250mg; sodium: 5mg; sugar: 18g.

Avocado Toast with Pumpkin Seeds

Preparation Time: 5 minutes   **Cooking Time:** 2 minutes   **Servings:** 1

INGREDIENTS:

- 1 slice whole grain bread
- 1/2 avocado, mashed
- 1 tbsp pumpkin seeds
- Pinch of sea salt

PREPARATION:

1. Toast the whole grain bread.
2. Spread mashed avocado on the toast.
3. Sprinkle with pumpkin seeds and sea salt.

Nutritional Information: calories: 250; carbohydrates: 20g; protein: 6g; fat: 18g; fiber: 7g; vitamins: E, B6; potassium: 400mg; sodium: 120mg; sugar: 2g.

Greek Yogurt with Flaxseeds and Fresh Berries

Preparation Time: 5 minutes   **Cooking Time:** 0 minutes   **Servings:** 1

INGREDIENTS:

- 1/2 cup Greek yogurt (dairy-free alternative if needed)
- 1 tbsp flaxseeds
- 1/4 cup fresh berries (blueberries, raspberries)

PREPARATION:

1. In a bowl, add Greek yogurt and top with flaxseeds and fresh berries.
2. Serve immediately.

Nutritional Information: calories: 150; carbohydrates: 15g; protein: 8g; fat: 5g; fiber: 4g; vitamins: C, K; potassium: 200mg; sodium: 55mg; sugar: 10g.

Edamame with Sea Salt

Preparation Time: 5 minutes   **Cooking Time:** 5 minutes   **Servings:** 2

INGREDIENTS:

- 1 cup edamame, in pods
- 1/2 tsp sea salt

PREPARATION:

1. Boil water and cook edamame for 5 minutes.
2. Drain and sprinkle with sea salt before serving.

Nutritional Information: calories: 160; carbohydrates: 14g; protein: 12g; fat: 6g; fiber: 5g; vitamins: C, K; potassium: 450mg; sodium: 230mg; sugar: 2g.

Chia Seed Energy Bars

Preparation Time: 10 minutes   **Cooking Time:** 0 minutes   **Servings:** 6

INGREDIENTS:

- 1 cup rolled oats (gluten-free)
- 2 tbsp chia seeds
- 1/4 cup almond butter
- 2 tbsp honey
- 1/4 cup dried cranberries

PREPARATION:

1. In a large bowl, mix oats, chia seeds, almond butter, honey, and dried cranberries.
2. Press the mixture into a lined baking dish.
3. Refrigerate for 30 minutes before cutting into bars.

Nutritional Information: calories: 210; carbohydrates: 28g; protein: 5g; fat: 10g; fiber: 6g; vitamins: E; potassium: 180mg; sodium: 30mg; sugar: 12g.

Carrot and Cucumber Sticks with Guacamole

Preparation Time: 10 minutes　　**Cooking Time:** 0 minutes　　**Servings:** 2

INGREDIENTS:

- 2 carrots, sliced into sticks
- 1 cucumber, sliced into sticks
- 1/2 cup guacamole

PREPARATION:

1. Arrange carrot and cucumber sticks on a plate.
2. Serve with guacamole on the side for dipping.

Nutritional Information: calories: 140; carbohydrates: 18g; protein: 3g; fat: 7g; fiber: 7g; vitamins: A, C; potassium: 400mg; sodium: 100mg; sugar: 8g.

Hard-Boiled Eggs with Avocado

Preparation Time: 5 minutes　　**Cooking Time:** 10 minutes　　**Servings:** 2

INGREDIENTS:

- 2 hard-boiled eggs
- 1/2 avocado, sliced
- Pinch of sea salt

PREPARATION:

1. Boil eggs for 10 minutes, then let them cool and peel.
2. Slice the eggs in half and serve with sliced avocado.
3. Sprinkle with sea salt.

Nutritional Information: calories: 220; carbohydrates: 6g; protein: 12g; fat: 17g; fiber: 5g; vitamins: E, B6; potassium: 420mg; sodium: 140mg; sugar: 1g.

Cottage Cheese with Pineapple and Walnuts

Preparation Time: 5 minutes　　**Cooking Time:** 0 minutes　　**Servings:** 1

INGREDIENTS:

- 1/2 cup cottage cheese (dairy-free alternative if needed)
- 1/4 cup pineapple chunks (fresh or canned in juice)
- 1 tbsp chopped walnuts

PREPARATION:

1. In a bowl, add cottage cheese.
2. Top with pineapple chunks and chopped walnuts.
3. Serve immediately.

Nutritional Information: calories: 190; carbohydrates: 15g; protein: 11g; fat: 10g; fiber: 2g; vitamins: C, D; potassium: 300mg; sodium: 300mg; sugar: 12g.

Roasted Almonds with Dark Chocolate Chips

Preparation Time: 5 minutes **Cooking Time:** 10 minutes **Servings:** 2

INGREDIENTS:

- 1/4 cup raw almonds
- 1 tbsp dark chocolate chips (70% cacao or higher)
- Pinch of sea salt

PREPARATION:

1. Preheat the oven to 350°F (175°C).
2. Spread almonds on a baking sheet and roast for 10 minutes.
3. Let the almonds cool, then mix with dark chocolate chips and a pinch of sea salt.

Nutritional Information: calories: 220; carbohydrates: 15g; protein: 6g; fat: 16g; fiber: 5g; vitamins: E; potassium: 250mg; sodium: 30mg; sugar: 8g.

Baked Zucchini Chips with Sea Salt

Preparation Time: 10 minutes **Cooking Time:** 30 minutes **Servings:** 2

INGREDIENTS:

- 1 large zucchini, thinly sliced
- 1 tbsp olive oil
- 1/4 tsp sea salt

PREPARATION:

1. Preheat the oven to 225°F (110°C).
2. Toss zucchini slices with olive oil and sea salt.
3. Spread the zucchini slices on a baking sheet in a single layer.
4. Bake for 30 minutes or until crispy.
5. Let cool before serving.

Nutritional Information: calories: 90; carbohydrates: 7g; protein: 2g; fat: 7g; fiber: 2g; vitamins: C; potassium: 280mg; sodium: 150mg; sugar: 4g.

Banana Slices with Peanut Butter and Chia Seeds

Preparation Time: 5 minutes   **Cooking Time:** 0 minutes   **Servings:** 1

INGREDIENTS:

- 1 medium banana, sliced
- 1 tbsp peanut butter
- 1 tsp chia seeds

PREPARATION:

1. Arrange banana slices on a plate.
2. Spread peanut butter on each slice.
3. Sprinkle with chia seeds and serve.

Nutritional Information: calories: 210; carbohydrates: 30g; protein: 5g; fat: 9g; fiber: 5g; vitamins: B6; potassium: 400mg; sodium: 50mg; sugar: 18g.

Smoked Salmon Roll-Ups with Cucumber and Cream Cheese

Preparation Time: 10 minutes   **Cooking Time:** 0 minutes   **Servings:** 2

INGREDIENTS:

- 4 slices smoked salmon
- 2 tbsp cream cheese (dairy-free alternative if needed)
- 1/2 cucumber, sliced into thin strips
- 1 tbsp fresh dill, chopped

PREPARATION:

1. Lay smoked salmon slices flat on a plate.
2. Spread cream cheese on each slice.
3. Add cucumber strips and sprinkle with fresh dill.
4. Roll up the salmon slices and serve.

Nutritional Information: calories: 150; carbohydrates: 4g; protein: 10g; fat: 10g; fiber: 1g; vitamins: A, D; potassium: 250mg; sodium: 350mg; sugar: 2g.

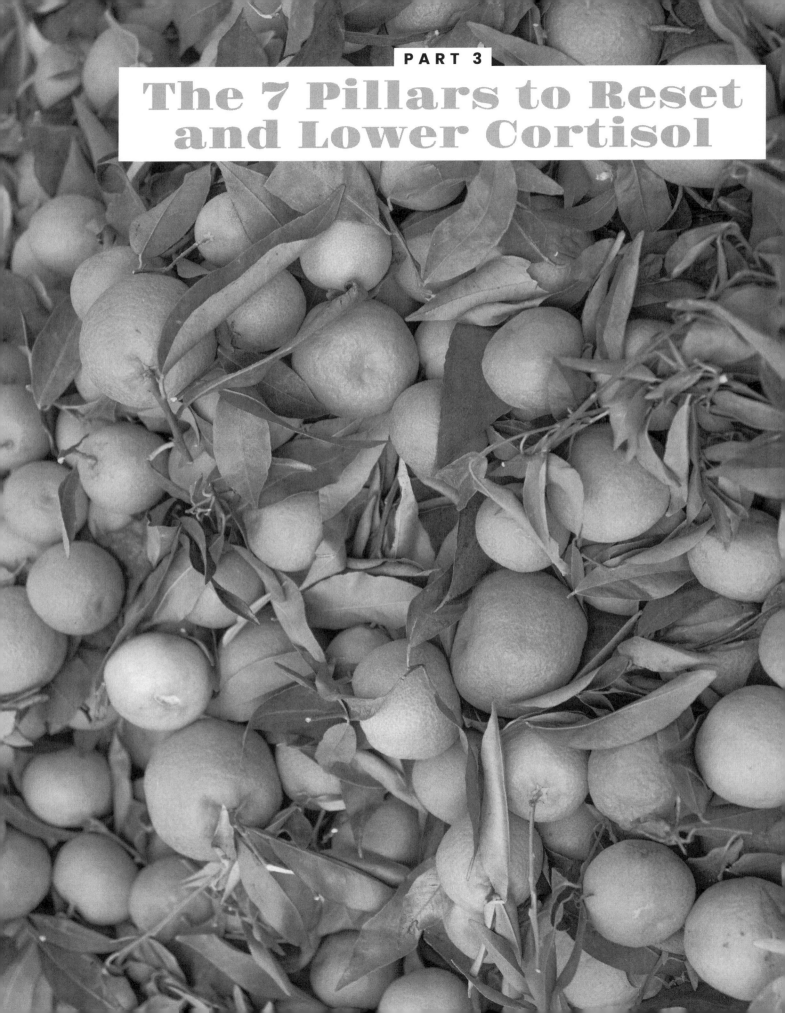

PART 3

The 7 Pillars to Reset and Lower Cortisol

CHAPTER 9

Nourishing Foods to Balance Cortisol

Key Nutrients That Support Cortisol Balance

When it comes to managing stress and maintaining balanced cortisol levels, what you eat plays a crucial role. Certain nutrients can directly influence how your body handles stress, promoting hormonal balance and supporting your adrenal glands in regulating cortisol production. By incorporating these key nutrients into your daily diet, you can help your body manage stress more effectively and prevent the damaging effects of chronically elevated cortisol. Below are the most important nutrients that support cortisol balance and how they work to keep you feeling calm, energized, and resilient.

1. Magnesium: The Calming Mineral

Magnesium is often referred to as nature's "calming" mineral, and for good reason. It plays a significant role in regulating your body's stress response and is essential for proper adrenal function. When you're stressed, your body depletes its magnesium stores more rapidly, which can lead to increased cortisol production.

- **How magnesium helps**: Magnesium helps regulate cortisol by inhibiting its release and promoting relaxation. It also supports GABA (gamma-aminobutyric acid), a neurotransmitter that promotes calmness and reduces anxiety.

- **Sources of magnesium**: Leafy greens (such as spinach and kale), almonds, cashews, avocados, and dark chocolate are all excellent sources of magnesium.

Incorporating magnesium-rich foods into your diet can have an immediate calming effect, helping you to feel more centered and less reactive to stressful situations.

2. Vitamin C: The Stress-Busting Antioxidant

Vitamin C is another essential nutrient for cortisol regulation. Known primarily as an immune booster, vitamin C also plays a key role in adrenal health. The adrenal glands, where cortisol is produced, contain some of the highest concentrations of vitamin C in the body. When you're under stress, your adrenal glands use up vitamin C more quickly, which can compromise their ability to regulate cortisol levels effectively.

- **How vitamin C helps**: Vitamin C helps to lower cortisol levels by supporting adrenal gland function and reducing oxidative stress, which can cause further cortisol production. It also enhances the production of dopamine and serotonin, two neurotransmitters that help improve mood and reduce stress.

- **Sources of vitamin C**: Citrus fruits (like oranges and grapefruits), strawberries, bell peppers, and broccoli are all rich in vitamin C.

Ensuring you get enough vitamin C is essential for keeping cortisol levels in check, especially during periods of heightened stress.

3. Omega-3 Fatty Acids: Reducing Inflammation and Cortisol

Omega-3 fatty acids are renowned for their anti-inflammatory properties, but they also play an important role in regulating cortisol levels. Chronic stress leads to inflammation in the body, which can further elevate cortisol. Omega-3s help combat this inflammation, promoting overall hormonal balance and reducing the stress response.

- **How omega-3s help**: Omega-3 fatty acids reduce the secretion of cortisol in response to stress and improve communication between cells, promoting a healthier stress response. They also support brain health, helping to stabilize mood and reduce anxiety.
- **Sources of omega-3s**: Fatty fish like salmon, sardines, and mackerel are excellent sources of omega-3s, as are flaxseeds, chia seeds, and walnuts for plant-based options.

By including omega-3s in your diet, you can reduce inflammation, support brain function, and help your body better manage stress-induced cortisol spikes.

4. B Vitamins: Supporting Adrenal Health

The family of B vitamins, particularly B5 (pantothenic acid) and B6, is essential for maintaining adrenal health and supporting the body's ability to cope with stress. When you're under chronic stress, your body uses up these vitamins more quickly, which can impair adrenal function and lead to higher cortisol levels.

- **How B vitamins help**: B5 is vital for adrenal hormone production, while B6 plays a key role in neurotransmitter synthesis, which regulates mood and stress. Together, these vitamins help balance cortisol levels by improving your body's stress resilience.
- **Sources of B vitamins**: Whole grains, eggs, poultry, fish, and legumes are all good sources of B vitamins, with B6 also found in bananas and avocados.

Getting enough B vitamins supports adrenal health, helping your body cope better with daily stress and keeping cortisol levels from spiraling out of control.

5. Zinc: A Critical Mineral for Stress Response

Zinc is often overlooked when discussing cortisol regulation, but it plays an important role in maintaining healthy cortisol levels. Zinc is required for the synthesis of various enzymes that regulate hormone production, including cortisol.

- **How zinc helps**: Zinc helps inhibit excessive cortisol release by supporting the immune system and reducing oxidative stress, which can trigger cortisol production. Zinc also improves the body's sensitivity to insulin, which can help balance blood sugar levels and reduce cortisol spikes.
- **Sources of zinc**: Oysters, beef, pumpkin seeds, and lentils are excellent sources of zinc.

Including zinc-rich foods in your diet helps protect your adrenal glands from becoming over-stressed and supports balanced cortisol production.

6. Adaptogens: Natural Cortisol Regulators

Adaptogens are natural substances found in certain plants and herbs that help the body adapt to stress and regulate cortisol. While not technically classified as nutrients, adaptogens like ashwagandha, rhodiola, and holy basil are powerful tools for cortisol balance.

- **How adaptogens help**: Adaptogens work by stabilizing the HPA (hypothalamic-pituitary-adrenal) axis, which regulates cortisol production. They help prevent cortisol from spiking during stressful situations and can also reduce the long-term effects of chronic stress.

- **Sources of adaptogens**: These can be found in herbal supplements, teas, or powders that can be added to smoothies or meals.

Incorporating adaptogens into your routine, particularly during high-stress periods, can provide significant support in keeping cortisol levels balanced.

By focusing on these key nutrients—magnesium, vitamin C, omega-3 fatty acids, B vitamins, zinc, and adaptogens—you can provide your body with the tools it needs to regulate cortisol effectively and manage stress. Balancing these nutrients through a varied, whole-food diet will help your adrenal glands function optimally, reduce the impact of chronic stress, and promote long-term well-being.

Top 5 Cortisol-Balancing Superfoods

Incorporating the right foods into your diet is a powerful way to support cortisol balance and reduce the impact of chronic stress on your body. Certain foods are rich in nutrients that directly influence cortisol regulation, helping your body to stay calm and resilient. Below are five superfoods that not only taste great but also provide the key nutrients needed to keep cortisol levels in check and support overall health.

1.   Avocados

Avocados are an excellent source of healthy fats, particularly **monounsaturated fats**, which help reduce inflammation and support adrenal health. They're also packed with **potassium**, a key nutrient that helps regulate blood pressure, especially during stressful times. Potassium helps counteract the effects of cortisol-induced hypertension, making it easier for your body to maintain balance during stressful periods.

- **Why they work**: Avocados are rich in B vitamins, particularly B5 (pantothenic acid), which is crucial for adrenal function and hormone balance.
- **How to incorporate**: Add avocado slices to salads, use them as a spread on toast, or blend them into smoothies for a creamy texture.

2.   Salmon

Salmon is one of the best sources of **omega-3 fatty acids**, which are known for their ability to lower inflammation and regulate cortisol. Omega-3s improve how your body handles stress by supporting brain health and reducing the secretion of cortisol during stressful moments.

- **Why it works**: Omega-3 fatty acids not only reduce cortisol but also enhance mood and brain function, making it easier to manage stress without turning to unhealthy coping mechanisms.
- **How to incorporate**: Enjoy grilled or baked salmon a couple of times a week, or add it to salads and grain bowls for a nutrient-dense meal.

3.   Dark Chocolate

Dark chocolate, in moderation, is not only a treat but also a powerful tool for lowering cortisol levels. Rich in **magnesium** and antioxidants, dark chocolate helps to relax the body and reduce stress by calming the nervous system. The flavonoids in dark chocolate are also known to improve mood and reduce the perception of stress.

- **Why it works**: Magnesium is essential for relaxation, and the antioxidants in dark chocolate combat oxidative stress, which can contribute to elevated cortisol.
- **How to incorporate**: Opt for dark chocolate that's at least 70% cacao. A small piece after meals can satisfy your sweet tooth while offering cortisol-lowering benefits.

4. Leafy Greens

Leafy greens such as **spinach, kale, and Swiss chard** are packed with **magnesium**, a mineral that helps regulate cortisol and promotes relaxation. These vegetables are also high in **B vitamins**, which are vital for energy production and adrenal function, making them essential for stress management.

- **Why they work**: The high magnesium content helps soothe the nervous system, and B vitamins support the body's ability to produce energy without increasing cortisol levels.
- **How to incorporate**: Add leafy greens to salads, stir-fries, or smoothies. They can also be steamed or sautéed as a side dish to complement any meal.

5. Blueberries

Blueberries are antioxidant powerhouses, particularly rich in **vitamin C**, which is crucial for adrenal function and lowering cortisol. Stress depletes vitamin C stores in the body, and consuming foods like blueberries helps replenish this essential nutrient, supporting immune health and cortisol regulation.

- **Why they work**: The high levels of antioxidants and vitamin C in blueberries help protect the body from the oxidative stress caused by elevated cortisol, while also boosting immune function.
- **How to incorporate**: Add blueberries to your breakfast, whether it's oatmeal, yogurt, or smoothies, or enjoy them as a snack throughout the day.

By incorporating these cortisol-balancing superfoods into your daily routine, you can help reduce stress, support adrenal health, and maintain a more balanced hormonal system, all while enjoying delicious, nutrient-packed meals.

Meal Prep Strategies for Busy Schedules

When life is hectic, eating healthy can feel like an overwhelming task, especially when you're trying to balance work, family, and personal commitments. But with a little planning, meal prepping can become your secret weapon for maintaining a cortisol-friendly diet without spending hours in the kitchen. By setting aside a small amount of time each week, you can ensure that you have nutritious, stress-reducing meals ready to go, even on your busiest days. Here are some simple, actionable meal prep strategies designed for busy women like you who need quick, healthy options to stay on track.

1. Plan Ahead with a Weekly Menu

Taking just 15-20 minutes each week to plan your meals will save you time and stress later. A weekly menu not only ensures you're eating balanced, cortisol-friendly meals, but it also prevents last-minute unhealthy choices.

- **How to do it**: Pick a day to plan your meals for the week. Focus on simple, nourishing recipes that incorporate cortisol-balancing nutrients like magnesium, omega-3s, and vitamin C. Once you've planned your meals, create a shopping list to ensure you have all the ingredients you need.
- **Bonus tip**: Consider rotating a few go-to recipes throughout the month to avoid decision fatigue and make the process even faster.

2. Batch Cooking for Multiple Meals

Batch cooking is one of the most efficient ways to meal prep, allowing you to prepare multiple meals in one session. This technique is perfect for busy schedules because it minimizes time in the kitchen while maximizing the number of ready-to-eat meals you have on hand.

- **How to do it**: Set aside a couple of hours once a week to cook large portions of staple foods, such as roasted vegetables, quinoa, grilled chicken, or a big pot of soup. Store these in individual portions that can be easily reheated or combined into different meals.
- **Bonus tip**: Invest in high-quality containers to keep your prepped meals fresh. Clear containers make it easier to see what you have on hand, reducing the mental effort of deciding what to eat.

3. Prep Snacks for Easy Grab-and-Go Options

Snacking is often where many people fall off track, especially when stress hits, and cravings for quick, unhealthy foods arise. By prepping cortisol-balancing snacks in advance, you can ensure that you always have healthy options available when hunger strikes.

- **How to do it**: Prep easy snacks like portioned-out nuts and seeds (rich in magnesium), boiled eggs, or containers of hummus with cut-up veggies. You can also make snack bars using oats, nuts, and dark chocolate for a quick energy boost that supports cortisol balance.
- **Bonus tip**: Use small containers or resealable bags to pre-portion snacks so you can grab them on the way out the door, saving time and avoiding overeating.

4. Cook Once, Eat Twice

This is a time-saving strategy that involves cooking larger dinners with the intention of eating the leftovers for lunch the next day. It reduces the time spent cooking multiple meals while ensuring that you have healthy, balanced options ready to go.

- **How to do it**: Double your dinner recipes and store the extra portions for lunch or even dinner later in the week. Dishes like stir-fries, soups, and casseroles work especially well for this strategy.
- **Bonus tip**: If you find yourself short on time in the mornings, pack your lunch immediately after dinner so it's ready to go the next day.

5. Simplify with One-Pot Meals

One-pot meals are a busy person's best friend. They require minimal prep, minimal cleanup, and are an efficient way to make a nutrient-dense meal that supports cortisol balance. These meals often include a combination of protein, healthy fats, and vegetables—all in one dish.

- **How to do it**: Opt for recipes like slow-cooker stews, sheet pan meals, or skillet dishes that cook everything together. This minimizes the time spent chopping, stirring, and cleaning up, while still delivering a balanced meal.
- **Bonus tip**: Slow-cooker and Instant Pot recipes are perfect for throwing everything together in the morning and coming home to a ready-to-eat dinner.

By incorporating these meal prep strategies into your routine, you can enjoy balanced, cortisol-friendly meals without the stress. Whether you have a few minutes each evening or prefer to batch cook once a week, these strategies will help you stay on track, even with a busy schedule.

CHAPTER 10

Stabilizing Blood Sugar for Weight Loss

Why Blood Sugar Spikes Trigger Stress

You've likely experienced that sudden burst of energy after eating something sweet, followed by a crash that leaves you feeling irritable and tired. This rollercoaster of blood sugar spikes and drops doesn't just affect your energy—it also triggers stress in your body, particularly through its impact on cortisol, the hormone responsible for regulating your stress response. Understanding why blood sugar spikes cause stress can help you make better choices that keep both your energy and stress levels stable throughout the day.

The Blood Sugar-Cortisol Connection

When you eat foods that are high in refined sugars or simple carbohydrates, your blood sugar rises quickly, leading to a spike in energy. While this might feel great at first, your body sees this spike as a problem and releases **insulin**, the hormone responsible for bringing your blood sugar back down to a safe level.

However, when insulin rapidly lowers your blood sugar, your body perceives the sudden drop as a threat to survival, triggering the release of cortisol to bring your blood sugar back up.

- **Cortisol's role**: Cortisol's primary job in this situation is to ensure you have enough glucose (sugar) in your bloodstream for energy. When blood sugar drops too low, cortisol is released to trigger the liver to produce more glucose and stabilize blood sugar levels. This process, though essential for survival, also puts your body in a state of stress.

- **Energy crashes**: As cortisol works to raise blood sugar after a drop, you may experience a crash in energy levels. This crash often leaves you feeling fatigued, anxious, or even shaky, which can increase stress and lead to cravings for quick energy sources like sugary snacks.

How Blood Sugar Spikes Increase Stress Hormones

Beyond cortisol, other stress hormones like **adrenaline** are also released when your blood sugar fluctuates wildly. This is because your body views these drastic changes in blood sugar as an emergency, triggering the same hormonal response you would have if you were in immediate physical danger.

- **Adrenaline's role**: Adrenaline, also known as the "fight-or-flight" hormone, is released along with cortisol to prepare your body for action. This surge in adrenaline can cause feelings of anxiety, rapid heartbeat, and restlessness, making you feel stressed even though there's no actual external threat.

- **Long-term effects**: Over time, these repeated blood sugar spikes and crashes can lead to chronic elevated cortisol levels, which not only makes weight loss difficult but also contributes to long-term health issues like insulin resistance, anxiety, and fatigue.

Cravings and the Cycle of Stress

One of the most frustrating aspects of blood sugar spikes is that they create a cycle of cravings and stress. After a blood sugar crash, your body craves quick sources of energy—typically foods high in sugar or refined carbohydrates. Giving in to these cravings results in another spike, followed by another crash, and the cycle repeats.

- **Increased cravings**: Each time your blood sugar drops, your body sends signals to the brain that it needs more sugar. This is why you might feel an intense craving for sweets or snacks when you're stressed or tired.

- **Emotional eating**: As cortisol and adrenaline levels rise, many people find themselves turning to food as a way to cope with the physical symptoms of stress, perpetuating the cycle of eating, crashing, and feeling stressed.

Managing Blood Sugar to Reduce Stress

The key to breaking this cycle is to **stabilize your blood sugar levels** throughout the day by eating balanced meals that include protein, healthy fats, and complex carbohydrates. This keeps your blood sugar steady, reduces the need for insulin spikes, and prevents cortisol from being released unnecessarily. By managing your blood sugar, you not only avoid energy crashes but also reduce the stress response in your body, leading to more balanced energy and a calmer mind.

Foods to Balance Blood Sugar and Curb Cravings

Balancing your blood sugar is essential not only for stabilizing energy but also for managing cravings that can derail your diet and weight loss efforts. When you eat foods that help keep your blood sugar steady, you prevent spikes and crashes that trigger cravings, particularly for sugary and refined carbohydrate-rich foods. By choosing nutrient-dense, slow-digesting foods, you can create a more balanced, controlled approach to eating that supports both your cortisol levels and your weight management goals.

1. Protein-Rich Foods

Protein is a key macronutrient when it comes to balancing blood sugar because it slows the absorption of carbohydrates and helps you feel fuller for longer. Including high-quality protein in each meal and snack can reduce hunger pangs and curb the desire for quick-fix sugary treats.

- **Why it works**: Protein stabilizes blood sugar by slowing down digestion, which helps prevent the rapid spikes and drops that lead to cravings. It also supports muscle repair and energy levels.

- **Examples**: Eggs, lean poultry, fish, tofu, lentils, and Greek yogurt are excellent protein sources. Including these in your meals helps keep blood sugar steady throughout the day.

2. Healthy Fats

Healthy fats, like those found in avocados, nuts, seeds, and olive oil, are critical for balancing blood sugar because they provide long-lasting energy without causing insulin spikes. Fats help slow the digestion of carbohydrates, which prevents rapid blood sugar fluctuations.

- **Why it works**: Fats keep you satiated for longer periods, reducing the need for constant snacking and minimizing sugar cravings.
- **Examples**: Incorporate foods like avocados, almonds, chia seeds, and olive oil into your meals. For instance, drizzle olive oil over a salad or snack on a handful of nuts to keep cravings at bay.

3. Fiber-Rich Vegetables

Non-starchy, fiber-rich vegetables like spinach, kale, broccoli, and bell peppers are fantastic for blood sugar regulation. Fiber slows the digestion of carbohydrates, which in turn helps regulate blood sugar and insulin levels. Additionally, high-fiber foods add bulk to your meals, promoting a feeling of fullness and preventing overeating.

- **Why it works**: Fiber prevents rapid glucose absorption into the bloodstream, helping to curb hunger and reduce cravings.
- **Examples**: Leafy greens, Brussels sprouts, and cucumbers are great choices. Aim to fill half your plate with non-starchy vegetables to add volume to meals without spiking blood sugar.

4. Whole Grains

Unlike refined grains, whole grains contain fiber, vitamins, and minerals that help stabilize blood sugar. They digest more slowly than processed carbohydrates, keeping your energy levels steady and curbing cravings for sugary snacks later in the day.

- **Why it works**: The fiber in whole grains slows digestion, preventing the quick release of glucose into the bloodstream that leads to sugar highs and subsequent crashes.
- **Examples**: Brown rice, quinoa, oats, and barley are excellent whole grain options. Try adding quinoa to salads or enjoy a bowl of oatmeal with chia seeds for breakfast.

5. Berries and Low-Glycemic Fruits

While many fruits contain natural sugars, low-glycemic options like berries are ideal for balancing blood sugar. Berries are rich in fiber, antioxidants, and essential vitamins while being relatively low in sugar, making them perfect for curbing sweet cravings without the blood sugar spikes.

- **Why it works**: Berries have a low glycemic index, which means they cause a slower rise in blood sugar compared to other fruits, helping prevent cravings and energy crashes.
- **Examples**: Blueberries, raspberries, and strawberries are great low-glycemic fruit options. Add them to yogurt or oatmeal for a sweet yet blood sugar-friendly snack.

Incorporating these foods into your diet will help balance your blood sugar, reduce cravings, and support your weight loss efforts. By prioritizing protein, healthy fats, fiber, whole grains, and low-glycemic fruits, you can take control of your blood sugar and curb the cycle of stress-induced cravings.

Simple Changes to Avoid Energy Crashes

Energy crashes—those moments when you suddenly feel fatigued, sluggish, or crave sugary snacks—are often the result of blood sugar imbalances. While it's tempting to reach for quick-fix foods like caffeine or sugary snacks, these only perpetuate the cycle of highs and lows. Fortunately, making a few simple changes to your diet and daily routine can help you stabilize your energy levels, keep your blood sugar balanced, and avoid those frustrating crashes.

1. Eat Balanced Meals with Protein, Fat, and Fiber

One of the most effective ways to avoid energy crashes is to make sure that every meal you eat contains a balance of **protein**, **healthy fats**, and **fiber**. These macronutrients slow down digestion, preventing rapid spikes in blood sugar followed by sudden drops.

- **Why it works**: Protein and healthy fats take longer to digest than carbohydrates, providing a steady source of energy. Fiber, especially from vegetables and whole grains, further slows the release of glucose into the bloodstream.
- **Simple change**: Instead of relying on a carb-heavy breakfast like cereal or toast, opt for scrambled eggs with avocado and spinach. For lunch, try a salad with grilled chicken, quinoa, and a drizzle of olive oil.

2. Snack Smart with High-Protein Options

Snacking strategically can help you maintain stable energy levels throughout the day, especially when hunger strikes between meals. The key is to avoid sugary snacks and refined carbohydrates, which cause blood sugar to spike and crash. Instead, choose high-protein snacks that keep you feeling full and energized for longer.

- **Why it works**: Protein-rich snacks help keep blood sugar steady by promoting slow digestion and preventing the sharp insulin spikes that lead to energy crashes.
- **Simple change**: Instead of grabbing a candy bar, try snacking on a handful of almonds, Greek yogurt, or a boiled egg. These snacks are rich in protein and healthy fats, which help maintain steady energy.

3. Avoid Skipping Meals

Skipping meals may seem like a convenient way to save time or cut calories, but it often backfires by leading to blood sugar drops and energy crashes later in the day. When your body goes too long without food, your blood sugar drops, triggering intense hunger and cravings for quick energy sources like sugar or processed carbs.

- **Why it works**: Eating regularly prevents large gaps between meals, ensuring that your blood sugar stays stable and your energy remains consistent.
- **Simple change**: Set a reminder to eat something every 3-4 hours, whether it's a meal or a healthy snack. This will prevent blood sugar dips and the energy crashes that follow.

4. Stay Hydrated Throughout the Day

Dehydration can mimic the symptoms of an energy crash, making you feel tired, unfocused, and sluggish. Often, what we perceive as hunger or fatigue is actually a sign that we need more water. Drinking enough water throughout the day helps your body maintain optimal function, including keeping blood sugar levels stable.

- **Why it works**: Staying hydrated supports your body's natural energy production and prevents the false sense of fatigue that dehydration can cause.
- **Simple change**: Keep a water bottle with you at all times and aim to drink about eight glasses of water a day. If plain water feels boring, try adding a slice of lemon or cucumber for a refreshing twist.

5. Include Complex Carbohydrates Instead of Refined Carbs

Not all carbohydrates are created equal. Refined carbs, like white bread and sugary snacks, cause rapid spikes in blood sugar followed by sharp crashes. To prevent this, focus on **complex carbohydrates** that are digested more slowly, providing sustained energy without the dramatic highs and lows.

- **Why it works**: Complex carbs, such as whole grains, sweet potatoes, and legumes, have a lower glycemic index, which means they release glucose more gradually into your bloodstream, preventing sudden energy dips.

- **Simple change**: Swap out refined carbs for whole grains—choose quinoa or brown rice instead of white rice, or replace white bread with whole grain alternatives.

By making these small but impactful changes, you can stabilize your blood sugar levels, avoid energy crashes, and maintain a steady flow of energy throughout your day. These adjustments not only improve how you feel but also support long-term weight management and stress reduction.

CHAPTER 11

Hydration and Cortisol Reduction

How Dehydration Increases Cortisol

Staying hydrated is about more than just quenching your thirst—it's essential for maintaining balanced cortisol levels and managing stress. When your body becomes dehydrated, it triggers a physiological response that can lead to elevated cortisol, the hormone responsible for regulating stress. This means that even mild dehydration can increase stress levels and contribute to a cycle of fatigue, anxiety, and stress-related health issues. Understanding how dehydration impacts cortisol is the first step toward using hydration as a tool for stress reduction.

The Link Between Hydration and Cortisol

Cortisol is produced by the adrenal glands and is released in response to both physical and emotional stress. While its primary role is to help the body cope with stress, chronic elevation of cortisol can lead to a range of negative health outcomes, including weight gain, anxiety, and sleep disturbances. Hydration plays a critical role in regulating cortisol production and maintaining balance in the body.

- **Fluid balance and adrenal function**: When your body is dehydrated, it perceives this as a form of physical stress. The adrenal glands respond by releasing cortisol to help manage the body's response to this stressor. In the short term, this response is helpful, but prolonged dehydration can lead to consistently elevated cortisol levels.

- **Increased cortisol in response to dehydration**: Research shows that even mild dehydration can lead to an increase in cortisol. This happens because dehydration puts extra strain on the body's systems, making it harder to regulate stress effectively. As cortisol levels rise, you may experience more frequent mood swings, anxiety, or difficulty concentrating.

Dehydration as a Physical Stressor

Your body needs water to perform essential functions such as regulating body temperature, transporting nutrients, and maintaining cellular balance. When you're dehydrated, these processes are disrupted, leading to physical stress that the body must compensate for. The release of cortisol is one way the body tries to manage this internal imbalance, but if dehydration persists, cortisol remains elevated, creating a cycle of stress that's difficult to break.

- **Physical fatigue**: Dehydration reduces blood volume, making it harder for your heart to pump oxygen and nutrients throughout the body. This leads to physical fatigue, which the body interprets as stress, further increasing cortisol production.

- **Cognitive impact**: Dehydration affects mental clarity and focus, leading to brain fog and difficulty concentrating. The stress associated with this cognitive decline causes the body to release more cortisol, exacerbating the cycle.

Hydration and the Stress Response

Ensuring that your body stays hydrated can help reduce cortisol levels and minimize the effects of stress. By keeping your body well-hydrated, you allow the adrenal glands to function properly and prevent unnecessary cortisol spikes.

- **Maintaining fluid balance**: Proper hydration helps regulate blood pressure, keeps your heart functioning efficiently, and allows the body to manage stress more effectively. With adequate water intake, your adrenal glands don't need to overproduce cortisol to handle the stress of dehydration.

- **Preventing cortisol spikes**: Drinking water consistently throughout the day helps prevent the small but frequent spikes in cortisol that occur when the body is under mild stress. Keeping a water bottle with you can remind you to stay hydrated and reduce the likelihood of dehydration-induced cortisol elevation.

By understanding the relationship between hydration and cortisol, you can use this knowledge to improve both your physical and mental well-being. Staying properly hydrated is a simple yet effective way to manage stress and support your body's natural ability to regulate cortisol levels.

Best Drinks for Lowering Cortisol

When it comes to managing cortisol levels and reducing stress, what you drink is just as important as what you eat. Certain beverages contain key nutrients and compounds that can help regulate cortisol production, promote relaxation, and support overall adrenal health. Incorporating these drinks into your daily routine can make a significant difference in how your body handles stress, helping you stay calm and balanced. Here are some of the best drinks for naturally lowering cortisol.

1. Green Tea

Green tea is rich in **L-theanine**, an amino acid that promotes relaxation without causing drowsiness. L-theanine works by influencing neurotransmitters in the brain, such as serotonin and dopamine, which help regulate mood and stress. Green tea also contains a modest amount of caffeine, which can provide a gentle energy boost without spiking cortisol levels like stronger caffeinated beverages might.

- **Why it works**: L-theanine in green tea reduces cortisol and helps promote a calm but alert state, making it ideal for reducing stress throughout the day.

- **How to enjoy**: Opt for a cup of green tea in the morning or early afternoon. If you're sensitive to caffeine, consider switching to **decaffeinated green tea** in the evening for similar cortisol-lowering effects.

2. Ashwagandha Tea

Ashwagandha is a well-known adaptogen, a type of herb that helps the body adapt to stress and balance cortisol levels. Studies have shown that ashwagandha significantly reduces cortisol levels and improves resilience to both physical and emotional stress. Drinking ashwagandha tea is an easy way to reap these benefits while also promoting relaxation.

- **Why it works**: Ashwagandha regulates the hypothalamic-pituitary-adrenal (HPA) axis, which is responsible for the body's stress response, helping to prevent cortisol spikes.

- **How to enjoy**: Look for pre-made ashwagandha tea or brew your own by steeping dried ashwagandha root in hot water. Drinking a cup in the evening can help you unwind after a stressful day.

3. Chamomile Tea

Chamomile is famous for its calming properties, and it's one of the best drinks to lower cortisol and promote restful sleep. Chamomile works as a natural **mild sedative**, helping reduce anxiety and tension, which in turn lowers cortisol levels. Its anti-inflammatory and antioxidant properties also support overall health and stress management.

- **Why it works**: Chamomile interacts with receptors in the brain that regulate mood, helping to ease anxiety and promote a sense of calm.
- **How to enjoy**: Drink a warm cup of chamomile tea an hour before bed to help lower cortisol levels and improve sleep quality.

4. Warm Lemon Water

Drinking warm water with freshly squeezed lemon is a simple and refreshing way to support adrenal function and reduce cortisol. Lemons are high in **vitamin C**, which is crucial for maintaining healthy cortisol levels, especially when you're under stress. Vitamin C helps lower cortisol and boost immune function, making this drink both stress-relieving and health-promoting.

- **Why it works**: Vitamin C plays a vital role in adrenal health, and warm lemon water provides a quick, easy source of this essential nutrient.
- **How to enjoy**: Start your day with a glass of warm water and lemon to support hydration and help your body manage stress from the get-go.

5. Coconut Water

Coconut water is a hydrating drink packed with **electrolytes** like potassium and magnesium, which are essential for reducing stress and supporting overall adrenal health. When you're stressed, your body tends to lose more electrolytes, especially through increased cortisol production. Drinking coconut water helps restore these nutrients and keeps you hydrated, which in turn helps lower cortisol levels.

- **Why it works**: The high levels of magnesium in coconut water help relax muscles and nerves, which reduces physical tension and lowers cortisol.
- **How to enjoy**: Drink coconut water throughout the day, especially if you're feeling fatigued or stressed. It's a great alternative to sugary sports drinks.

Incorporating these drinks into your daily routine can make a big difference in managing your cortisol levels. Whether you choose a calming herbal tea or a refreshing glass of coconut water, each of these beverages offers unique benefits that help your body handle stress and promote balance.

Anti-Cortisol Beverage Recipes

Incorporating anti-cortisol beverages into your daily routine is a simple and enjoyable way to manage stress naturally. These recipes combine ingredients that are rich in nutrients known to reduce cortisol, improve mood, and support adrenal health. Each of these drinks can help you stay hydrated, calm your nervous system, and promote balance in your body. Here are some easy-to-make, delicious anti-cortisol beverages that you can enjoy throughout the day.

1. Ashwagandha & Almond Milk Latte

Ashwagandha is a powerful adaptogen known for its cortisol-lowering properties. This soothing latte combines ashwagandha with creamy almond milk for a stress-relieving beverage that's perfect for unwinding in the evening.

Ingredients:

- 1 teaspoon **ashwagandha powder**
- 1 cup **unsweetened almond milk**
- 1 teaspoon **honey** or maple syrup (optional)
- 1/2 teaspoon **cinnamon**
- 1/4 teaspoon **vanilla extract**

Instructions:

1. Warm the almond milk in a small saucepan over medium heat until hot but not boiling.
2. Whisk in the ashwagandha powder, honey, cinnamon, and vanilla extract.
3. Pour into a mug and enjoy as a calming nighttime drink.

Why it works: Ashwagandha helps regulate the body's stress response, while the almond milk provides healthy fats to keep you satiated and calm.

2. Chamomile & Lavender Iced Tea

Chamomile and lavender are both known for their relaxing properties, making this iced tea a perfect anti-cortisol beverage to sip during a busy day. Chamomile reduces anxiety and tension, while lavender promotes relaxation and reduces stress-induced cortisol spikes.

Ingredients:

- 2 **chamomile tea bags**
- 1 teaspoon **dried lavender** (or 1 drop of lavender essential oil, food-grade)
- 2 cups **boiling water**
- 1 teaspoon **honey** (optional)
- Ice cubes

Instructions:

1. Steep the chamomile tea bags and dried lavender in boiling water for 5-7 minutes.
2. Remove the tea bags and strain out the lavender. Add honey if desired.
3. Let the tea cool and then pour it over a glass of ice.

Why it works: Chamomile and lavender work together to reduce cortisol levels by promoting relaxation and soothing the nervous system.

3. Coconut Water & Berry Smoothie

Coconut water is a great source of electrolytes like magnesium and potassium, which help lower cortisol and reduce physical stress on the body. Paired with antioxidant-rich berries, this smoothie helps combat oxidative stress while keeping you hydrated and energized.

Ingredients:

- 1 cup **coconut water**
- 1/2 cup **frozen blueberries**
- 1/2 cup **frozen raspberries**
- 1 tablespoon **chia seeds**
- 1 tablespoon **flaxseeds**

Instructions:

1. Add all the ingredients to a blender and blend until smooth.
2. Pour into a glass and enjoy this refreshing, cortisol-balancing smoothie.

Why it works: Coconut water replenishes electrolytes and supports adrenal health, while the antioxidants in the berries fight oxidative stress that can lead to cortisol elevation.

4. Warm Lemon & Ginger Elixir

This warm lemon and ginger drink is packed with **vitamin C**, an essential nutrient for regulating cortisol levels. Ginger adds anti-inflammatory benefits, while the lemon supports detoxification and hydration, making this drink a perfect way to start your day.

Ingredients:

- 1 cup **warm water**
- Juice of 1 **lemon**
- 1 teaspoon **grated fresh ginger**
- 1 teaspoon **honey** (optional)

Instructions:

1. In a mug, combine the warm water, lemon juice, and grated ginger.
2. Stir well and add honey for sweetness if desired.

Why it works: Vitamin C from the lemon helps reduce cortisol, while ginger supports digestion and further reduces stress-induced inflammation.

5. Golden Milk (Turmeric Latte)

Turmeric contains **curcumin**, a compound with powerful anti-inflammatory properties that also helps lower cortisol levels. This golden milk recipe combines turmeric with warming spices and coconut milk for a soothing, anti-inflammatory drink.

Ingredients:

- 1 cup **unsweetened coconut milk**
- 1 teaspoon **turmeric powder**
- 1/4 teaspoon **cinnamon**
- 1/4 teaspoon **ginger powder**
- 1 teaspoon **honey** (optional)
- Pinch of **black pepper** (to enhance turmeric absorption)

Instructions:

1. Heat the coconut milk in a saucepan over medium heat.
2. Add turmeric, cinnamon, ginger, and black pepper. Whisk until well combined.
3. Stir in honey, if using. Pour into a mug and enjoy this warming, anti-cortisol beverage.

Why it works: Turmeric's anti-inflammatory properties help reduce cortisol, while the coconut milk provides healthy fats that support adrenal function and overall relaxation.

These simple anti-cortisol beverage recipes can easily be added to your daily routine, helping you stay calm and balanced while supporting your body's natural stress response.

CHAPTER 12

Restorative Movement and Exercise

Why Intense Exercise May Increase Stress

While exercise is often heralded as a powerful stress reliever, not all types of exercise produce the same effects on the body. In fact, for some individuals, particularly those who are already managing high stress levels, intense exercise can lead to increased cortisol production and exacerbate feelings of stress and anxiety. Understanding why this occurs is crucial for selecting the right type of exercise that supports rather than undermines your mental health.

The Body's Stress Response

Intense exercise, such as high-intensity interval training (HIIT) or heavy weightlifting, places a significant physical demand on the body. When you engage in this type of strenuous activity, your body perceives it as a form of stress. In response, the body releases cortisol and adrenaline—hormones designed to help you cope with physical challenges.

- **Fight or flight response**: The increase in these stress hormones triggers the "fight or flight" response, preparing your body to either confront or flee from a perceived threat. While this response is beneficial in short bursts, prolonged activation can lead to chronic stress.

- **Cortisol spikes**: Intense workouts can lead to spikes in cortisol, especially if the workouts are frequent and not balanced with adequate recovery. High cortisol levels can contribute to increased anxiety, mood swings, and fatigue, counteracting the intended benefits of exercising.

Overtraining Syndrome

For individuals who push their limits regularly without allowing adequate recovery time, the risk of developing **overtraining syndrome** increases. Overtraining occurs when the body is unable to recover from the physical demands placed upon it, leading to a variety of negative symptoms.

- **Symptoms of overtraining**: These can include persistent fatigue, decreased performance, insomnia, and increased susceptibility to illness. Overtraining places undue stress on the body, leading to elevated cortisol levels and further exacerbating feelings of stress.

- **Hormonal imbalance**: Chronic overtraining can disrupt hormonal balance, not only affecting cortisol but also impacting other hormones like insulin, estrogen, and testosterone, further complicating the body's stress response.

It's important to recognize that everyone's body reacts differently to exercise. While some individuals thrive on high-intensity workouts and experience stress relief, others may find that such activities leave them feeling drained and more stressed.

- **Personal thresholds**: Factors like fitness level, mental health status, and personal stress levels can all influence how your body responds to intense exercise. A workout that feels invigorating to one person may feel overwhelming to another.

- **Listening to your body**: It's essential to listen to your body's signals. If you notice increased fatigue, irritability, or heightened stress following intense workouts, it may be time to reassess your exercise routine.

Finding Balance in Your Exercise Routine

To manage stress effectively while still reaping the benefits of exercise, finding a balance between intense workouts and low-stress activities is vital. Incorporating a variety of workout types can help maintain hormonal balance while keeping exercise enjoyable.

- **Mixing it up**: Combine high-intensity sessions with lower-impact activities such as yoga, Pilates, or walking. These forms of exercise promote relaxation, flexibility, and mindfulness, helping to mitigate the stress response triggered by intense workouts.

- **Focus on recovery**: Prioritize recovery strategies such as rest days, adequate sleep, and hydration to support your body in managing stress and maintaining energy levels.

By understanding how intense exercise can sometimes increase stress, you can make informed choices about your fitness routine that support your overall well-being.

Low-Stress Workouts to Lower Cortisol

In today's fast-paced world, finding effective ways to manage stress is essential for overall well-being. While intense workouts can sometimes elevate cortisol levels, low-stress exercises provide a gentle yet powerful way to lower cortisol and promote relaxation. These types of workouts not only help reduce stress but also enhance mood, improve flexibility, and increase energy levels. Here's a look at some of the best low-stress workouts to incorporate into your routine.

1. Yoga

Yoga is one of the most effective low-stress workouts available. By combining physical postures, breath control, and mindfulness, yoga helps calm the nervous system, reduce cortisol levels, and enhance mental clarity.

- **Benefits**: Studies have shown that practicing yoga regularly can lead to significant reductions in cortisol levels and anxiety. The focus on deep breathing promotes relaxation and encourages the body to enter a state of calm.

- **How to start**: You can begin with simple poses such as Child's Pose, Cat-Cow, or Forward Fold, gradually incorporating more complex postures as you become comfortable. Many online platforms offer beginner-friendly yoga classes that you can follow at home.

2. Walking

Walking is a low-impact activity that is accessible to everyone. It's an excellent way to get moving without putting your body under significant stress. Taking regular walks can also provide a mental break from daily responsibilities.

- **Benefits**: Walking promotes the release of endorphins, the body's natural mood boosters, and has been linked to lower cortisol levels. The rhythmic nature of walking helps calm the mind and reduce anxiety.
- **How to start**: Aim for at least 30 minutes of brisk walking most days of the week. You can break this up into shorter walks if needed. Consider walking in nature, as the calming effects of the outdoors can enhance the benefits of this simple exercise.

3. Tai Chi

Tai Chi is a form of martial art that focuses on slow, flowing movements and deep breathing. This gentle practice is often referred to as "meditation in motion," making it an excellent choice for reducing stress.

- **Benefits**: Research indicates that practicing Tai Chi can significantly lower cortisol levels and enhance emotional well-being. The focus on breath and movement encourages relaxation and mindfulness.
- **How to start**: Look for local Tai Chi classes or online tutorials that provide instruction on basic movements. Many communities offer free outdoor classes in parks, especially during the warmer months.

4. Pilates

Pilates is another low-stress workout that focuses on core strength, flexibility, and body awareness. This method emphasizes controlled movements and proper alignment, making it an effective way to relieve tension and improve posture.

- **Benefits**: Pilates promotes relaxation through deep breathing and controlled movements, which can help reduce cortisol levels and stress. Additionally, it strengthens muscles without the intensity of traditional strength training.
- **How to start**: You can find beginner Pilates classes in your area or follow along with online videos that guide you through foundational exercises.

5. Gentle Stretching

Incorporating gentle stretching into your daily routine is a fantastic way to relieve tension, improve flexibility, and calm the mind. Stretching helps release muscle tightness and promotes relaxation, making it an ideal low-stress activity.

- **Benefits**: Regular stretching can reduce cortisol levels and improve circulation, which enhances overall physical and mental well-being.
- **How to start**: Spend 10-15 minutes each day stretching major muscle groups, focusing on areas that feel tight. Include stretches for the neck, shoulders, back, and legs.

6. Dancing

Dancing can be a joyful way to express yourself while keeping stress levels low. Whether it's a formal dance class or simply grooving to your favorite tunes at home, dancing is an excellent form of low-stress exercise.

- **Benefits**: Dancing releases endorphins, boosts mood, and fosters a sense of community and connection, all of which contribute to lowering cortisol levels.
- **How to start**: Put on your favorite music and dance freely in your living room, or join a local dance class that matches your interests, whether it's Zumba, ballroom, or hip-hop.

Incorporating these low-stress workouts into your routine can significantly reduce cortisol levels and enhance your overall sense of well-being. By focusing on gentle, restorative movements, you can cultivate a healthier response to stress, supporting both your physical and mental health in the long run.

20-Minute Daily Exercise Plan

Finding time for exercise can be a challenge, especially with a busy schedule. However, you don't need long, intense sessions to see results or lower your cortisol levels. A simple, consistent 20-minute daily exercise plan can help you manage stress, support weight loss, and improve your overall well-being. This plan incorporates gentle, restorative movements designed to lower cortisol, boost energy, and promote relaxation—all without overwhelming your body or increasing stress.

Warm-Up (2-3 Minutes)

Starting with a gentle warm-up helps to prepare your body for exercise by gradually increasing your heart rate and loosening your muscles.

- **Movement**: Start with 2-3 minutes of light cardio, such as walking in place, arm circles, or shoulder rolls.
- **Focus**: Concentrate on your breathing. Inhale deeply through your nose and exhale slowly, which signals your body to stay calm while preparing for movement.

Dynamic Stretching (3-5 Minutes)

Dynamic stretching helps to improve flexibility and range of motion, making it easier to perform the exercises ahead without strain. This also helps to prevent injury and keeps muscles relaxed.

- **Hip circles**: Stand with feet hip-width apart. Slowly rotate your hips in a circular motion for 10 seconds in one direction, then switch.
- **Leg swings**: Hold onto a wall or chair for balance. Swing one leg forward and backward in a controlled motion, repeating 10-12 times on each leg.
- **Arm reaches**: Extend your arms above your head, interlace your fingers, and stretch gently to each side for 15 seconds.

Core Strengthening (5 Minutes)

Strengthening your core helps improve posture, reduces tension in the body, and supports overall body movement. These exercises are low-stress and help engage the abdominal muscles without overworking your system.

- **Cat-Cow Pose** (1 minute): On your hands and knees, alternate between arching your back (cow pose) and rounding it (cat pose) in rhythm with your breathing. This movement gently warms up the spine while engaging your core.
- **Bird-Dog Pose** (1 minute): From a tabletop position, extend your right arm forward and your left leg back. Hold for a few seconds, then switch sides. Repeat for 1 minute.
- **Plank Hold** (2 minutes): Get into a plank position on your forearms or hands. Hold for 30 seconds, rest, and repeat for another 30 seconds, focusing on core engagement and steady breathing.

Lower Body and Flexibility (7 Minutes)

Focusing on the lower body can help relieve tension, improve circulation, and promote strength without causing cortisol spikes.

- **Bodyweight Squats** (2 minutes): Stand with feet hip-width apart. Lower into a squat position, keeping your weight in your heels, then return to standing. Aim for 12–15 reps.
- **Lunges** (2 minutes): Step one foot forward into a lunge, then return to standing. Switch legs, repeating 10–12 times on each side.
- **Seated Forward Fold** (1 minute): Sit on the floor with your legs extended in front of you. Slowly fold forward, reaching toward your toes, and hold for 30 seconds to stretch the hamstrings.

Cool Down and Breathing (3 Minutes)

Cooling down is essential to lower your heart rate, reduce cortisol levels, and help your muscles relax after exercise. Focus on deep, slow breathing as you move through gentle stretches.

- **Child's Pose** (1 minute): Kneel on the floor, sitting back on your heels, and stretch your arms forward, bringing your forehead to the floor. Breathe deeply and relax into the pose.
- **Supine Twist** (1 minute): Lie on your back, bring one knee toward your chest, and gently twist your body by bringing your knee across to the opposite side. Hold for 30 seconds on each side.
- **Deep Breathing** (1 minute): Finish by lying on your back or sitting in a comfortable position. Close your eyes and take deep, slow breaths. Inhale for 4 counts, hold for 4 counts, and exhale for 6 counts. This helps signal your body to relax and reduce cortisol.

Improving Sleep for Stress Recovery

How Poor Sleep Raises Cortisol

Sleep is an essential part of the body's recovery process, allowing your brain and body to rest, repair, and reset for the day ahead. However, when sleep is disrupted or insufficient, it can trigger a cascade of stress responses, leading to elevated cortisol levels. Cortisol, the body's main stress hormone, plays a crucial role in regulating energy, metabolism, and the body's response to stress, but when it's consistently elevated due to poor sleep, it can negatively impact your health.

The Sleep-Cortisol Connection

Cortisol follows a natural rhythm, peaking in the morning to help you wake up and slowly decreasing throughout the day to its lowest levels at night. This pattern, known as the **circadian rhythm**, is closely tied to your sleep-wake cycle. When you get enough quality sleep, cortisol follows this rhythm, helping you feel alert in the morning and calm in the evening.

However, when sleep is poor or interrupted, this delicate rhythm is disrupted:

- **Increased cortisol during the night**: If you struggle with falling or staying asleep, your body may interpret this as a stress signal. In response, cortisol levels rise, making it even harder to fall asleep or stay asleep, creating a vicious cycle.

- **Difficulty waking up**: Without restorative sleep, cortisol levels may remain abnormally high in the evening and not peak as they should in the morning. This can make waking up a challenge, leaving you feeling groggy and unrefreshed.

Chronic Sleep Deprivation and Cortisol

Chronic sleep deprivation leads to consistently elevated cortisol levels, which has several negative effects on your body and mind:

- **Increased stress response**: Sleep deprivation heightens your body's stress response, leading to the release of more cortisol throughout the day. This makes you more susceptible to feeling anxious, irritable, or overwhelmed by even minor stressors.

- **Impact on metabolism**: High cortisol levels affect your metabolism, leading to increased appetite and cravings for high-sugar or high-fat foods. This is why sleep-deprived individuals often struggle with weight gain, particularly around the abdomen.

- **Impaired cognitive function**: Elevated cortisol also impairs cognitive function, making it harder to concentrate, remember things, and manage emotions. This mental fog can further contribute to stress, creating a loop of poor sleep and high cortisol.

The Role of REM Sleep

Rapid Eye Movement (REM) sleep is a critical stage of the sleep cycle where the brain processes emotions, consolidates memories, and regulates stress hormones. When you don't get enough REM sleep, cortisol levels may remain elevated, contributing to heightened stress.

- **Sleep fragmentation**: Interrupted sleep prevents the body from completing the full sleep cycle, including REM sleep. The less REM sleep you get, the more cortisol remains in your system the next day.

- **Emotional regulation**: REM sleep plays a vital role in regulating emotions. Without enough REM, you may feel more emotionally reactive or less able to handle stress, leading to a further increase in cortisol production.

How Poor Sleep Impacts Your Body

The cumulative effect of elevated cortisol due to poor sleep can lead to several health issues, including:

- **Immune system suppression**: High cortisol levels over time can suppress the immune system, making you more vulnerable to infections and illnesses.

- **Increased inflammation**: Cortisol is meant to regulate inflammation, but when it's chronically elevated, it can lead to increased inflammation in the body, contributing to conditions like cardiovascular disease and diabetes.

- **Disrupted hormone balance**: Prolonged sleep deprivation can also disrupt other hormone levels, including insulin and ghrelin (the hunger hormone), further complicating weight management and overall health.

By recognizing the connection between poor sleep and elevated cortisol, you can take steps to prioritize restful, uninterrupted sleep, helping to break the cycle of stress and support better overall health.

Simple Tips for Better Sleep

Improving your sleep quality is one of the most effective ways to lower cortisol levels and enhance your overall well-being. Sleep is when your body and brain recover from daily stress, but for many people, achieving a restful night's sleep can be challenging. Whether you're dealing with stress, anxiety, or a busy schedule, adopting a few simple habits can help you get the restorative sleep you need. Here are some practical tips for improving your sleep quality and creating an environment that supports relaxation and recovery.

1. Create a Consistent Sleep Schedule

One of the best ways to improve sleep is by sticking to a regular sleep schedule. Going to bed and waking up at the same time every day helps regulate your body's internal clock, known as the **circadian rhythm**. This rhythm governs your sleep-wake cycle and is closely tied to cortisol levels.

- **How to do it**: Set a consistent bedtime and wake-up time, even on weekends. Aim for 7-9 hours of sleep each night to allow your body enough time to recover.

- **Why it works**: A consistent routine stabilizes your body's natural cortisol pattern, promoting easier sleep onset and better sleep quality.

2. Limit Screen Time Before Bed

The blue light emitted by screens from phones, tablets, and computers can interfere with your body's production of **melatonin**, the hormone responsible for making you feel sleepy. Too much screen time before bed delays melatonin release, making it harder to fall asleep.

- **How to do it**: Avoid screens for at least one hour before bedtime. If you need to use your devices in the evening, consider using blue light-blocking glasses or enabling the night mode on your phone or computer.
- **Why it works**: Reducing blue light exposure helps your body naturally wind down and allows melatonin to do its job, making it easier to fall asleep and stay asleep.

3. Create a Relaxing Bedtime Routine

A calming bedtime routine signals to your body that it's time to wind down and prepares your mind for sleep. This helps reduce stress, lower cortisol levels, and create a smooth transition into sleep.

- **How to do it**: Incorporate relaxing activities such as reading, journaling, deep breathing exercises, or listening to calming music before bed. You can also take a warm bath to help relax your muscles.
- **Why it works**: Engaging in relaxing activities helps shift your body from a state of alertness to rest, lowering cortisol levels and easing your mind into sleep.

4. Optimize Your Sleep Environment

Your sleep environment plays a significant role in how well you sleep. A comfortable, quiet, and cool bedroom can make it easier to fall asleep and stay asleep.

- **How to do it**: Keep your bedroom cool, between 60-67°F (15-20°C), and ensure it's dark and quiet. Consider using blackout curtains, earplugs, or a white noise machine if necessary.
- **Why it works**: A dark and quiet environment supports melatonin production, while a cool temperature promotes deeper, uninterrupted sleep.

5. Be Mindful of Caffeine and Alcohol Intake

Caffeine and alcohol can significantly interfere with your sleep cycle. While caffeine is a stimulant that can keep you awake, alcohol may disrupt your sleep later in the night, causing you to wake up frequently.

- **How to do it**: Avoid caffeine in the afternoon and limit alcohol intake in the evening. Both substances can raise cortisol levels and prevent deep, restful sleep.
- **Why it works**: Reducing caffeine and alcohol helps keep your body's cortisol levels balanced, supporting better sleep quality.

6. Incorporate Gentle Movement or Stretching

Engaging in light physical activity such as stretching or yoga before bed can help relieve tension in your body and lower cortisol. Gentle movement promotes relaxation and prepares your muscles for rest.

- **How to do it**: Spend 5-10 minutes doing gentle stretches or a relaxing yoga routine to release physical tension. Focus on deep, slow breathing to further promote relaxation.
- **Why it works**: Gentle movement reduces stress, promotes blood flow, and helps your body shift into a calm state, making it easier to fall asleep.

By incorporating these simple tips into your daily routine, you can improve the quality of your sleep, lower cortisol levels, and enhance your body's ability to recover from stress.

How to Stop Waking Up at 2 a.m.

Waking up in the middle of the night—especially around 2 a.m.—is a common problem for many people, and it can significantly disrupt your sleep quality and stress recovery. This pattern of interrupted sleep often stems from a combination of factors, including elevated cortisol levels, poor sleep habits, and underlying stress or anxiety. The good news is that with a few adjustments to your routine, you can minimize these nighttime awakenings and get back to restorative sleep.

1. Regulate Blood Sugar Before Bed

One of the most common reasons for waking up at 2 a.m. is blood sugar instability. If your blood sugar drops too low during the night, your body may release cortisol and adrenaline to restore glucose levels, which can wake you up.

- **How to fix it**: Eat a small, balanced snack before bed that includes protein and healthy fats to stabilize blood sugar levels. For example, a handful of almonds or a slice of turkey with avocado can help prevent blood sugar dips during the night.
- **Why it works**: Stabilizing blood sugar helps maintain steady energy levels throughout the night, preventing the cortisol spike that can cause early awakenings.

2. Reduce Evening Stress Levels

High stress and anxiety can lead to increased cortisol production, especially in the evening. When cortisol levels remain elevated at night, it can disrupt your sleep cycle, making it more likely that you'll wake up in the early hours of the morning.

- **How to fix it**: Incorporate calming practices into your evening routine, such as deep breathing exercises, meditation, or gentle yoga. These activities help activate the **parasympathetic nervous system**, signaling your body that it's time to wind down.
- **Why it works**: Reducing stress before bed lowers cortisol levels, promoting deeper, uninterrupted sleep and reducing the likelihood of waking up at 2 a.m.

3. Limit Fluid Intake Before Bed

Waking up to use the bathroom is another common reason for nighttime disruptions. Drinking too much liquid close to bedtime can lead to more frequent trips to the bathroom, which may contribute to 2 a.m. awakenings.

- **How to fix it**: Stop drinking fluids at least 1-2 hours before bed to minimize nighttime bathroom trips. If you feel thirsty before bed, take small sips rather than large gulps.
- **Why it works**: Limiting fluid intake allows your body to stay asleep without the need for middle-of-the-night interruptions, ensuring a more restful night.

4. Keep Your Sleep Environment Cool and Dark

Your body temperature naturally drops during the night, which is essential for promoting deep sleep. However, if your bedroom is too warm, this can interfere with your body's ability to reach the optimal temperature for sleep, causing you to wake up.

- **How to fix it**: Keep your bedroom temperature between 60-67°F (15-20°C) and ensure your room is as dark as possible. Use blackout curtains or a sleep mask to block any ambient light, which can disrupt your sleep cycle.
- **Why it works**: A cool, dark environment helps regulate your body's natural sleep-wake cycle and lowers cortisol levels, making it easier to stay asleep throughout the night.

5. Establish a Pre-Bedtime Routine

A consistent pre-bedtime routine can signal to your body that it's time to sleep, reducing the likelihood of waking up during the night. If you regularly wake up at 2 a.m., your body may need a stronger signal to recognize when it's time for deep, uninterrupted sleep.

- **How to fix it**: Start your bedtime routine 30-60 minutes before you plan to sleep. Incorporate relaxing activities such as reading, listening to calming music, or taking a warm bath. Avoid stimulating activities like watching TV or scrolling through your phone, as these can keep your brain too active.

- **Why it works**: A consistent routine helps reinforce your body's circadian rhythm and tells your brain when it's time to rest, reducing middle-of-the-night awakenings.

6. Consider Melatonin Supplements

For some people, waking up at 2 a.m. may be linked to an imbalance in melatonin, the hormone responsible for regulating sleep. If your body isn't producing enough melatonin at night, your sleep cycle may be disrupted.

- **How to fix it**: Consider taking a low-dose melatonin supplement (around 0.5 to 3 mg) about 30 minutes before bed. Consult with a healthcare provider before starting any supplements.

- **Why it works**: Melatonin helps regulate your sleep-wake cycle and supports your body's natural rhythm, reducing the likelihood of waking up during the night.

By incorporating these strategies into your daily routine, you can address the common causes of 2 a.m. awakenings, improve your sleep quality, and support cortisol regulation for better stress recovery.

CHAPTER 14

Gut Health and Its Role in Cortisol Balance

The Gut-Cortisol Connection

Your gut plays a far more significant role in your overall health than you might realize, and it's deeply connected to how your body handles stress. The **gut-cortisol connection** refers to the relationship between your gut microbiome—the collection of bacteria, fungi, and other microorganisms in your digestive system—and the regulation of cortisol, your primary stress hormone. When your gut is healthy, it helps to balance cortisol levels, but when it's out of balance, it can lead to increased stress and higher cortisol production, creating a cycle that's tough to break.

How the Gut Affects Cortisol Levels

The gut and the brain are in constant communication via what is known as the **gut-brain axis**. This bi-directional pathway allows signals to flow back and forth between the gut and the brain, influencing various bodily functions, including mood, stress response, and digestion.

- **Microbiome and cortisol regulation**: A healthy gut microbiome helps regulate the hypothalamic-pituitary-adrenal (HPA) axis, which controls cortisol production. When the microbiome is balanced, the signals sent to the brain are calming, helping to keep cortisol levels in check. However, when the gut is imbalanced—often due to poor diet, stress, or antibiotics—it can trigger inflammation and stress signals that lead to increased cortisol production.

- **Leaky gut and cortisol**: Another way the gut influences cortisol levels is through **intestinal permeability**, commonly known as leaky gut. When the gut lining becomes compromised, harmful bacteria and toxins can enter the bloodstream, triggering an immune response. This process increases inflammation throughout the body and leads to elevated cortisol levels as the body attempts to fight off perceived threats.

How Cortisol Impacts Gut Health

Just as the gut influences cortisol levels, cortisol can also impact the health of your gut. When you're under chronic stress, and cortisol is consistently elevated, it can have several negative effects on the digestive system:

- **Reduced diversity of gut bacteria**: High cortisol levels can reduce the diversity of beneficial bacteria in the gut, leading to dysbiosis—an imbalance of harmful and good bacteria. This imbalance further exacerbates inflammation and stress, worsening the gut's ability to regulate cortisol.

- **Slowed digestion**: Cortisol diverts energy away from non-essential functions like digestion during times of stress. Over time, this can lead to issues like indigestion, bloating, and even irritable bowel syndrome (IBS).
- **Impact on gut motility**: Elevated cortisol levels can disrupt gut motility—the speed at which food moves through the digestive system. This can result in either constipation or diarrhea, further contributing to discomfort and stress.

The Role of Inflammation in the Gut-Cortisol Cycle

Inflammation is a key player in the gut-cortisol connection. Chronic inflammation in the gut—often triggered by a poor diet, stress, or an unhealthy microbiome—can lead to increased production of **pro-inflammatory cytokines**, which signal to the brain that the body is under stress. This, in turn, raises cortisol levels as the body attempts to mitigate the inflammation.

- **Inflammation and stress**: The more inflammation there is in your gut, the more likely you are to experience elevated cortisol levels, creating a vicious cycle. High cortisol increases inflammation, and inflammation raises cortisol—making it essential to address gut health to break this cycle.
- **Gut-healing strategies**: Reducing gut inflammation through diet, probiotics, and stress management is one of the most effective ways to lower cortisol and restore balance in the gut.

The Importance of a Healthy Gut for Cortisol Balance

Maintaining a healthy gut is crucial for managing cortisol levels and reducing stress. By nurturing your gut microbiome through diet and lifestyle changes, you can support better digestion, improve your body's stress response, and lower cortisol levels naturally.

- **Probiotics and prebiotics**: Incorporating foods rich in probiotics (like yogurt, kefir, and fermented vegetables) and prebiotics (like garlic, onions, and bananas) helps feed the beneficial bacteria in your gut, promoting a balanced microbiome that supports cortisol regulation.
- **Anti-inflammatory foods**: Eating a diet rich in anti-inflammatory foods—such as leafy greens, berries, and fatty fish—helps reduce gut inflammation and lower cortisol levels.

Understanding the gut-cortisol connection empowers you to make choices that support both your mental and physical well-being. A healthy gut is a powerful tool in managing stress and achieving hormonal balance.

Foods and Probiotics to Heal Your Gut

A healthy gut is essential for regulating cortisol levels and reducing stress. Your gut microbiome— the trillions of microorganisms living in your digestive system—plays a crucial role in how your body manages stress and inflammation. When your gut is out of balance, it can lead to elevated cortisol, poor digestion, and increased stress. However, by incorporating specific foods and probiotics into your diet, you can support your gut's health, improve digestion, and help your body naturally lower cortisol levels.

The Role of Probiotics in Gut Healing

Probiotics are live microorganisms that provide a wide range of health benefits, particularly for gut health. These beneficial bacteria help restore balance in the gut microbiome by promoting the growth of good bacteria and reducing harmful bacteria. By replenishing the gut with probiotics, you can improve digestion, reduce inflammation, and support cortisol balance.

- **How probiotics work**: Probiotics enhance gut barrier function, which prevents harmful substances from leaking into the bloodstream. This helps reduce inflammation and the body's stress response, lowering cortisol production.
- **Sources of probiotics**: Probiotics can be found in fermented foods and supplements. Regularly consuming probiotic-rich foods helps maintain a diverse and healthy gut microbiome.

Top Probiotic-Rich Foods for Gut Health

Incorporating probiotic-rich foods into your daily diet is one of the easiest ways to heal your gut and support cortisol regulation. Here are some of the best options to consider:

- **Yogurt**: Yogurt made with live active cultures is a well-known source of probiotics. It contains strains like **Lactobacillus** and **Bifidobacterium**, which help balance the gut microbiome. Choose plain, unsweetened yogurt to avoid excess sugar, which can promote inflammation and disrupt gut health.
- **Kefir**: Kefir is a fermented milk drink that's packed with probiotics. It contains a wider variety of beneficial bacteria compared to yogurt, making it an excellent choice for gut healing. It's also rich in vitamins and minerals that support overall gut health.
- **Sauerkraut**: Sauerkraut is fermented cabbage, and it's loaded with probiotics, especially **Lactobacillus**. The fermentation process increases the levels of beneficial bacteria, which help restore gut balance. Additionally, sauerkraut is high in fiber, which is important for feeding the good bacteria in your gut.

Prebiotic Foods: Fuel for Good Bacteria

While probiotics introduce beneficial bacteria into your gut, **prebiotics** provide the food these bacteria need to thrive. Prebiotic foods contain fibers that pass through the digestive system undigested, feeding the good bacteria in your gut and helping them grow.

- **Garlic**: Garlic is a potent prebiotic that contains **inulin**, a type of fiber that stimulates the growth of beneficial gut bacteria. Adding garlic to your meals can boost gut health and support the microbiome.
- **Onions**: Onions are another excellent source of inulin and act as fuel for the good bacteria in your gut. They also have natural anti-inflammatory properties, making them a great addition to a gut-healing diet.
- **Bananas**: Bananas, particularly when slightly underripe, are rich in prebiotic fibers like **fructooligosaccharides**. These fibers promote the growth of beneficial bacteria and help improve digestion, contributing to a healthier gut environment.

Combining Probiotics and Prebiotics

To maximize gut healing, it's important to combine probiotic and prebiotic foods in your diet. This combination creates a symbiotic relationship in your gut, where probiotics are nourished and supported by prebiotics, leading to a healthier and more balanced microbiome.

- **Example of a symbiotic meal**: Pair probiotic-rich yogurt with a banana or add garlic and onions to a dish with sauerkraut. These combinations will provide both beneficial bacteria and the fuel they need to thrive, promoting better gut health and cortisol balance.

In addition to yogurt and kefir, other fermented foods can introduce a wide variety of probiotics into your diet:

- **Kimchi**: A traditional Korean dish made from fermented vegetables, kimchi is rich in probiotics that support digestion and reduce inflammation.
- **Miso**: Miso is a fermented soybean paste used in soups and sauces. It contains beneficial bacteria that support gut health and improve immune function.

By incorporating these probiotic and prebiotic-rich foods into your daily routine, you can heal your gut, reduce inflammation, and naturally lower cortisol levels. A healthy gut leads to a more balanced stress response and better overall well-being.

Three Foods to Improve Gut Health This Week

Improving your gut health doesn't require complicated dietary changes—just a few small adjustments can make a significant difference. By incorporating specific gut-healing foods into your meals this week, you can start to see improvements in digestion, reduce inflammation, and support cortisol balance. Here are three key foods that are simple to add to your diet and will help strengthen your gut microbiome, leading to better overall health and lower stress levels.

1.   Sauerkraut: A Probiotic Powerhouse

Sauerkraut is one of the best foods for improving gut health, thanks to its high content of natural probiotics. Made by fermenting cabbage, sauerkraut is packed with beneficial bacteria, particularly **Lactobacillus**, which helps balance the gut microbiome and support digestion.

- **Why it works**: Fermentation not only preserves the cabbage but also enhances its nutritional value. The probiotics in sauerkraut help restore balance to the gut by promoting the growth of healthy bacteria, which can reduce inflammation and improve the body's ability to manage stress. This is especially important for lowering cortisol levels.
- **How to include it**: Add a spoonful of sauerkraut to salads, sandwiches, or as a side dish with your meals. Make sure to choose raw, unpasteurized sauerkraut, as pasteurization kills the beneficial bacteria.

2.   Chia Seeds: Fiber for a Healthy Gut

Chia seeds are an excellent source of dietary fiber, particularly **soluble fiber**, which helps promote gut health by feeding the beneficial bacteria in your digestive system. This fiber acts as a prebiotic, supporting the growth of good bacteria and aiding in digestion.

- **Why it works**: Chia seeds absorb water and form a gel-like substance in the stomach, which helps slow digestion and maintain steady blood sugar levels. This process helps prevent the spikes and crashes in blood sugar that can trigger stress and elevate cortisol. Additionally, the fiber in chia seeds keeps your digestive system running smoothly and supports a healthy gut barrier.
- **How to include it**: Sprinkle chia seeds on yogurt, add them to smoothies, or make a chia seed pudding for breakfast. You can also add them to salads or soups for an extra fiber boost.

3.   Bone Broth: A Gut-Healing Superfood

Bone broth has gained popularity as a gut-healing food, and for good reason. It's rich in **collagen** and **gelatin**, which help repair and strengthen the gut lining, reducing the risk of leaky gut syndrome. When the gut lining is compromised, harmful substances can leak into the bloodstream, triggering inflammation and increasing cortisol production.

- **Why it works**: The collagen and amino acids found in bone broth, such as **glutamine**, help heal the intestinal lining and reduce inflammation. This supports the overall health of the gut and helps lower cortisol by reducing the body's stress response to inflammation.

- **How to include it**: Sip a cup of warm bone broth as a snack or use it as a base for soups and stews. You can also add it to grains, like quinoa or rice, for extra flavor and gut-healing benefits.

How These Foods Support Cortisol Balance

Each of these foods plays a unique role in improving gut health, which in turn helps regulate cortisol levels. By supporting a healthy microbiome with probiotic-rich sauerkraut, feeding beneficial bacteria with fiber-packed chia seeds, and healing the gut lining with bone broth, you create a foundation for better digestion and a balanced stress response. Regularly consuming these foods will not only improve your gut health but also support your body's ability to manage stress more effectively.

CHAPTER 15

Using Adaptogens and Nutrients to Fight Stress

The Power of Adaptogens in Lowering Cortisol

Adaptogens are powerful herbs and plants that help your body adapt to stress and maintain balance, particularly by regulating cortisol levels. For centuries, adaptogens have been used in traditional medicine to enhance the body's resilience to physical, emotional, and environmental stressors. In today's world, where chronic stress is often unavoidable, adaptogens offer a natural, effective way to support your body's stress response and lower cortisol, the hormone responsible for managing stress.

How Adaptogens Work to Balance Cortisol

Adaptogens work by interacting with the hypothalamic-pituitary-adrenal (HPA) axis, which controls the production of cortisol and other stress hormones. When you're under stress, your adrenal glands release cortisol as part of the body's fight-or-flight response. While this is helpful in short bursts, chronic stress can lead to consistently elevated cortisol levels, which can cause fatigue, weight gain, anxiety, and other health issues.

- **Stress modulation**: Adaptogens help balance cortisol by enhancing the body's ability to adapt to stress. They do this by regulating the HPA axis, ensuring that cortisol is produced in appropriate amounts—high when you need it (like during intense physical activity) and low when you need to rest and recover.

- **Improving resilience**: Regular use of adaptogens can increase your resilience to stress over time, meaning that you'll respond better to stressful situations with less cortisol production and fewer negative effects on your health.

Key Adaptogens for Lowering Cortisol

Several adaptogens are particularly effective at reducing cortisol and supporting overall stress relief. Here are a few that stand out for their cortisol-lowering properties:

- **Ashwagandha**: One of the most well-known adaptogens, ashwagandha has been shown in numerous studies to significantly reduce cortisol levels. It helps regulate the HPA axis and is especially effective for those dealing with chronic stress or anxiety. Ashwagandha not only lowers cortisol but also improves sleep quality, which is crucial for stress recovery.

- **Rhodiola Rosea**: This adaptogen is known for its ability to boost mental clarity and physical endurance, making it an excellent choice for combating the fatigue associated with high cortisol levels. Rhodiola works by balancing the stress response and reducing cortisol spikes caused by intense mental or physical exertion.

- **Holy Basil (Tulsi)**: Holy basil is revered for its calming properties and its ability to lower cortisol levels. It has anti-inflammatory and antioxidant benefits that help protect the body from the long-term effects of stress. Holy basil is often used to reduce anxiety and improve mood, making it a great adaptogen for emotional stress.
- **Eleuthero (Siberian Ginseng)**: Eleuthero supports the adrenal glands by enhancing energy levels and reducing the impact of stress. It helps lower cortisol in response to both physical and mental stressors, making it a versatile adaptogen for those experiencing stress-induced fatigue.

The Benefits of Lowering Cortisol with Adaptogens

Using adaptogens to manage stress and lower cortisol levels offers a range of benefits for both your mental and physical health:

- **Improved energy and mood**: By keeping cortisol levels in check, adaptogens help reduce feelings of fatigue and irritability, allowing you to feel more balanced and energized throughout the day.
- **Better sleep**: High cortisol levels can interfere with sleep, leading to insomnia or poor-quality rest. Adaptogens like ashwagandha promote better sleep by calming the body's stress response and encouraging deeper relaxation.
- **Weight management**: Chronically elevated cortisol can lead to weight gain, particularly around the abdomen. Lowering cortisol through adaptogens helps the body better regulate metabolism and reduces stress-induced cravings for unhealthy foods.
- **Enhanced immune function**: Chronic stress and elevated cortisol can weaken the immune system, making you more susceptible to illness. Adaptogens not only lower cortisol but also support immune health, helping to protect against infections and inflammation.

Incorporating adaptogens into your routine can be a powerful tool for managing stress naturally. These herbs work gently yet effectively to lower cortisol, support adrenal health, and improve your body's resilience to stress, helping you feel more balanced and in control even in the face of daily challenges.

Essential Vitamins and Minerals for Stress Relief

When it comes to managing stress and supporting cortisol balance, certain vitamins and minerals play a crucial role in helping your body cope with the demands of daily life. These essential nutrients not only help regulate stress hormones but also support the overall health of the nervous system, promote energy production, and reduce inflammation. By ensuring you're getting enough of these key nutrients, you can enhance your body's ability to manage stress and lower cortisol levels naturally.

1. Vitamin C: The Stress-Busting Antioxidant

Vitamin C is well-known for its immune-boosting properties, but it also plays a vital role in managing stress. This powerful antioxidant helps regulate cortisol levels by supporting the adrenal glands, which are responsible for cortisol production.

- **Why it works**: During times of stress, your body uses up vitamin C quickly. Ensuring adequate levels of vitamin C helps your adrenal glands function properly, preventing excessive cortisol production. It also reduces oxidative stress, which can contribute to inflammation and worsen the body's stress response.

- **Sources**: Citrus fruits (oranges, lemons), bell peppers, strawberries, and broccoli are excellent sources of vitamin C.

2. Magnesium: The Relaxation Mineral

Magnesium is often referred to as the "relaxation mineral" because of its ability to calm the nervous system and promote relaxation. It is essential for regulating the body's stress response and maintaining balanced cortisol levels.

- **Why it works**: Magnesium helps regulate neurotransmitters like serotonin and GABA, which promote a sense of calm. It also plays a role in reducing cortisol by supporting the HPA axis, the system that controls the body's response to stress. Magnesium deficiency has been linked to increased anxiety and stress, making it a key nutrient for stress management.
- **Sources**: Dark leafy greens (spinach, kale), almonds, pumpkin seeds, and avocados are rich in magnesium.

3. B Vitamins: Energy and Stress Management

The B vitamins, particularly B6, B12, and folate, are essential for energy production, brain function, and mood regulation. They help the body convert food into energy and support the nervous system, making them crucial for stress management.

- **Why it works**: B vitamins, especially B6, help in the synthesis of neurotransmitters like serotonin and dopamine, which are essential for mood regulation. They also support the adrenal glands in producing and regulating cortisol. A deficiency in B vitamins can lead to fatigue, irritability, and increased stress.
- **Sources**: Whole grains, eggs, poultry, and leafy greens are great sources of B vitamins.

4. Zinc: Supporting the Adrenal Glands

Zinc is a trace mineral that plays a key role in supporting the immune system and helping the body cope with stress. It is also important for maintaining healthy adrenal function, which in turn helps regulate cortisol levels.

- **Why it works**: Zinc helps modulate the body's response to stress by supporting the adrenal glands and reducing inflammation. It also promotes the proper function of the immune system, which can become compromised when cortisol levels are chronically elevated.
- **Sources**: Foods rich in zinc include oysters, beef, pumpkin seeds, and lentils.

5. Omega-3 Fatty Acids: Anti-Inflammatory Support

Omega-3 fatty acids are essential fats that reduce inflammation and support brain health. They also help regulate the body's stress response by reducing the impact of cortisol on the body.

- **Why it works**: Chronic stress can lead to increased inflammation, which worsens cortisol imbalances. Omega-3s help reduce this inflammation and support the nervous system by improving communication between brain cells. This, in turn, reduces cortisol production and helps manage stress more effectively.
- **Sources**: Fatty fish (salmon, mackerel), flaxseeds, chia seeds, and walnuts are rich in omega-3 fatty acids.

6. Vitamin D: The Sunshine Vitamin for Stress

Vitamin D is known for its role in bone health, but it also plays a significant role in regulating mood and reducing stress. Low levels of vitamin D have been linked to increased stress, anxiety, and depression.

- **Why it works**: Vitamin D helps regulate the production of serotonin, a neurotransmitter that promotes a positive mood and reduces stress. It also supports the immune system, helping to reduce the body's stress response. Inadequate levels of vitamin D can lead to increased cortisol production and worsen the effects of stress.

- **Sources**: Sunlight exposure is the best source of vitamin D, but it can also be found in fortified foods like milk, eggs, and fatty fish.

By ensuring you get enough of these essential vitamins and minerals, you can support your body's natural stress response, lower cortisol levels, and enhance overall well-being. Incorporating these nutrients into your diet will help you feel more balanced, energized, and resilient in the face of daily stressors.

How to Incorporate Adaptogens into Your Routine

Adding adaptogens to your daily routine can significantly help in managing stress and lowering cortisol levels. These herbs work gently with your body, providing natural support for your adrenal glands and helping you build resilience to both physical and mental stress. The key to incorporating adaptogens successfully is consistency and finding what works best for your lifestyle. Here's how you can easily add adaptogens into your routine to experience their full benefits.

1. Choose the Right Adaptogen for Your Needs

Different adaptogens serve various purposes, so it's important to select the ones that align with your stress-relief goals and overall wellness needs. Here's a quick guide to help you choose:

- **Ashwagandha**: Ideal if you're dealing with chronic stress, anxiety, or fatigue. It's known for lowering cortisol and promoting better sleep.

- **Rhodiola Rosea**: Best for boosting energy and mental clarity, particularly if you experience stress-related fatigue.

- **Holy Basil (Tulsi)**: Excellent for managing emotional stress and promoting a calm, focused mind.

- **Maca**: A great option for balancing hormones and improving mood, particularly if stress is affecting your energy and libido.

2. Start with Small Doses and Build Gradually

When introducing adaptogens into your routine, start with small doses to see how your body responds. Adaptogens are generally safe, but everyone's body reacts differently, so it's important to monitor how you feel.

- **How to start**: Begin with the lowest recommended dose, typically 500 mg to 1 gram per day, and gradually increase it as needed over a couple of weeks.

- **Why it works**: Starting small helps you gauge how the adaptogen affects your energy, mood, and stress levels, allowing you to adjust the dosage accordingly.

3. Incorporate Adaptogens Into Your Morning or Evening Routine

Adaptogens can easily be added to your morning or evening routines, depending on their effects. Some adaptogens, like Rhodiola or Maca, are energizing and best taken in the morning, while others like Ashwagandha or Holy Basil promote relaxation and are better suited for the evening.

- **Morning routine**: Add Rhodiola or Maca to your morning smoothie or a glass of water for an energy boost that will help you power through the day without causing stress-related fatigue.

- **Evening routine**: Incorporate Ashwagandha or Holy Basil into your evening routine by mixing them into herbal teas or taking them in supplement form after dinner to promote calmness and prepare your body for restful sleep.

4. Try Adaptogenic Teas and Lattes

One of the simplest ways to incorporate adaptogens into your daily routine is by drinking adaptogenic teas or lattes. These beverages offer an easy, enjoyable way to consume your daily dose of adaptogens.

- **How to make it**: Mix powdered adaptogens like Ashwagandha or Reishi into warm almond milk with a dash of cinnamon and honey for a soothing adaptogenic latte. Alternatively, brew herbal teas infused with adaptogens like Holy Basil or Ginseng for a calming, stress-relieving drink.

- **Why it works**: Adaptogenic teas and lattes make it simple to consume adaptogens regularly, and you can easily adjust the strength to suit your taste and wellness needs.

5. Use Adaptogen Supplements

If you prefer a more straightforward approach, adaptogen supplements are available in capsule, powder, or tincture form. These supplements are easy to integrate into your daily supplement routine and can provide consistent benefits without requiring extra preparation.

- **How to use it**: Take adaptogen supplements with food to improve absorption and reduce any potential digestive discomfort. You can also mix powdered adaptogens into smoothies, yogurt, or soups for added convenience.

- **Why it works**: Supplements offer a measured, reliable dose of adaptogens, making it easier to track how much you're taking and ensuring you're getting consistent results.

6. Combine Adaptogens with Other Healthy Habits

For the best results, combine adaptogens with other stress-relief techniques and healthy habits like regular exercise, a balanced diet, and mindfulness practices. Adaptogens work synergistically with these lifestyle changes to enhance your body's ability to manage stress and lower cortisol levels.

- **How to combine**: Pair your adaptogens with a morning meditation session or gentle yoga practice to amplify their calming effects. Alternatively, take adaptogens post-workout to support recovery and reduce physical stress.

- **Why it works**: Incorporating adaptogens into a holistic approach to stress management helps you maximize their benefits while supporting overall well-being.

By following these simple steps, you can seamlessly incorporate adaptogens into your daily routine and enjoy their powerful effects on stress, energy, and cortisol balance. With consistency and mindful use, adaptogens can become an essential tool in your wellness journey, helping you navigate life's stressors with greater resilience and calm.

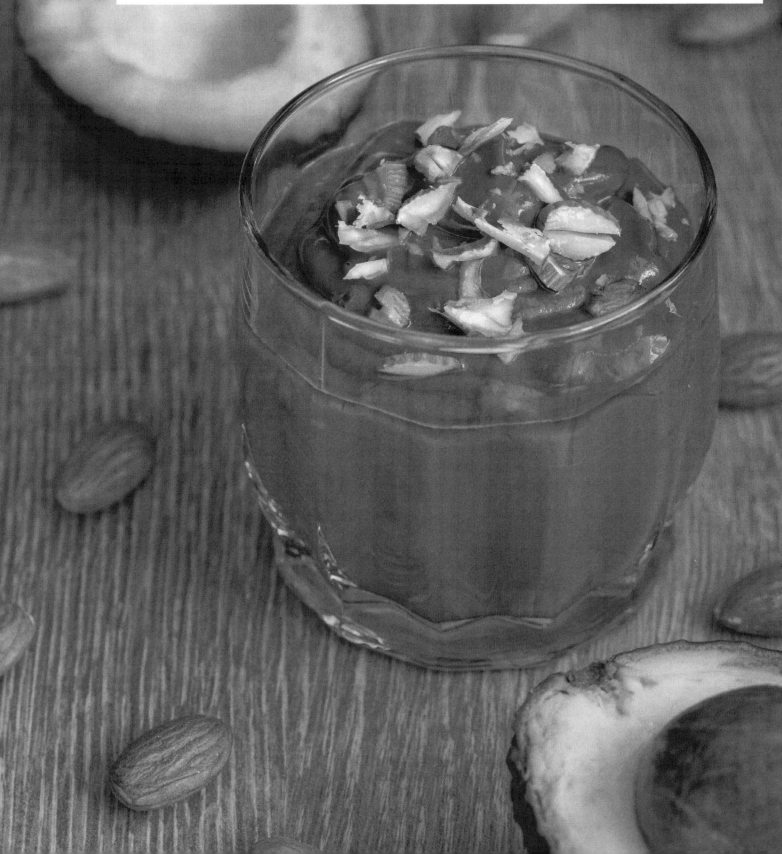

PART 4

The 28-Day Cortisol Detox Program

CHAPTER 16

Week 1 - Reset and Recharge

Cutting Out Stress-Triggering Foods

The foods you eat can have a profound effect on your stress levels and overall well-being. Some foods can trigger an increase in cortisol production and inflammation, which can lead to higher stress, fatigue, and even weight gain. To reset and recharge your body, it's essential to cut out these stress-triggering foods, especially during the first week of your journey to improved health and vitality. Eliminating or reducing these foods will help lower cortisol levels, reduce inflammation, and provide a solid foundation for the next phases of your detox plan.

1. Refined Sugars and Processed Carbohydrates

One of the most significant stress-triggering culprits in the modern diet is refined sugar and processed carbohydrates. These foods cause blood sugar spikes, which lead to a rapid release of insulin. When your blood sugar crashes, your body releases cortisol to restore balance, causing additional stress on your system.

- **Why it's harmful**: Frequent spikes and crashes in blood sugar lead to a cycle of increased cortisol production, which can cause anxiety, irritability, and cravings for more sugar.
- **How to cut it out**: Avoid sugary snacks, sodas, white bread, pastries, and other refined carbs. Replace them with whole grains, fruits, and vegetables, which provide more stable energy without the blood sugar rollercoaster.

2. Caffeine

Caffeine is a known stimulant that can disrupt sleep patterns and elevate cortisol levels, especially when consumed in excess. While a small amount of caffeine may help you feel alert, too much can lead to jitteriness, anxiety, and heightened stress.

- **Why it's harmful**: Caffeine stimulates the adrenal glands to release more cortisol, which can increase stress and disrupt your natural energy rhythms. Over time, this can lead to adrenal fatigue, where your body struggles to produce the necessary hormones to manage stress.
- **How to cut it out**: Limit your caffeine intake by reducing coffee, energy drinks, and caffeinated sodas. If quitting cold turkey feels too extreme, start by replacing one cup of coffee with a calming herbal tea, such as chamomile or peppermint.

3. Alcohol

Alcohol is often seen as a way to unwind, but it can actually increase stress on the body by disrupting sleep, impairing digestion, and raising cortisol levels. Regular alcohol consumption can lead to imbalances in blood sugar and create inflammation, both of which contribute to increased stress.

- **Why it's harmful**: Alcohol interferes with the body's ability to regulate cortisol and negatively impacts liver function, which is crucial for detoxification. It can also disrupt sleep, further compounding stress and fatigue.

- **How to cut it out**: During the first week of your reset, it's essential to eliminate alcohol entirely. Replace alcoholic beverages with sparkling water infused with lemon or mint to stay hydrated and refreshed.

4. Trans Fats and Highly Processed Oils

Trans fats and highly processed vegetable oils (such as soybean, corn, and canola oil) contribute to inflammation in the body, which can increase cortisol production. These unhealthy fats are commonly found in fried foods, packaged snacks, and fast foods.

- **Why it's harmful**: Inflammation caused by trans fats and processed oils forces the body to produce more cortisol to manage the inflammatory response. Over time, this can lead to chronic stress, weight gain, and heart health issues.
- **How to cut it out**: Avoid fried foods, fast foods, and processed snacks that contain hydrogenated oils. Instead, cook with healthy fats like olive oil, coconut oil, or avocado oil, which have anti-inflammatory properties.

5. Artificial Sweeteners and Additives

Artificial sweeteners, preservatives, and additives found in many processed foods can have a negative effect on gut health, which is closely tied to stress regulation. Disrupting the gut microbiome can lead to increased cortisol levels and a weakened immune system.

- **Why it's harmful**: Artificial sweeteners like aspartame and sucralose can disrupt the balance of good bacteria in the gut, leading to inflammation and stress hormone imbalances. These additives can also cause cravings for sugary foods, further perpetuating the cycle of cortisol spikes.
- **How to cut it out**: Read food labels carefully and avoid products with artificial sweeteners, preservatives, and additives. Opt for whole, unprocessed foods that are free of these hidden stress triggers.

By cutting out these stress-triggering foods during the first week of your reset, you'll be taking a crucial step toward lowering cortisol levels and improving your overall health. This foundational change will help you feel more balanced, energized, and ready to take on the next phases of your detox journey.

Meal Plan: Anti-Inflammatory Recipes to Start Your Journey

As you embark on your stress reset journey, a critical part of reducing cortisol and promoting overall well-being is following an anti-inflammatory meal plan. These recipes are designed to nourish your body while minimizing inflammation, a key factor that contributes to elevated cortisol levels and stress. In this first week, you'll focus on whole, nutrient-dense foods that support your body's natural ability to heal and recover from the damaging effects of chronic stress.

The goal of this anti-inflammatory meal plan is to provide you with easy, delicious recipes that are packed with vitamins, minerals, and antioxidants to fight inflammation, balance your hormones, and boost energy levels.

Key Principles of an Anti-Inflammatory Diet

To start, it's important to understand the foundational elements of an anti-inflammatory diet:

- **Whole foods**: Focus on whole, unprocessed foods like fruits, vegetables, lean proteins, and healthy fats. These foods are rich in the nutrients your body needs to fight inflammation.
- **Healthy fats**: Include plenty of omega-3 fatty acids, which are known to reduce inflammation. Sources include fatty fish like salmon, as well as plant-based options like flaxseeds and chia seeds.
- **Antioxidant-rich vegetables**: Dark leafy greens, colorful vegetables, and berries are all high in antioxidants that help neutralize free radicals and reduce oxidative stress.
- **Spices and herbs**: Incorporate anti-inflammatory spices like turmeric, ginger, and garlic, which help regulate cortisol levels and combat inflammation.

Sample Anti-Inflammatory Meal Plan

Here's a sample meal plan to help you reset and recharge during your first week. These meals are designed to be simple, flavorful, and packed with nutrients that support your body's ability to manage stress.

Breakfast Options

- **Overnight Chia Pudding with Berries**: Soak chia seeds in almond milk overnight and top with fresh berries and a drizzle of honey. Chia seeds are rich in fiber and omega-3s, helping to keep your gut healthy and reduce inflammation.
- **Avocado Toast with Poached Egg**: Spread mashed avocado on whole grain toast, top with a poached egg, and sprinkle with chili flakes for a boost of healthy fats and protein. This combo helps balance blood sugar and keeps cortisol in check.

Lunch Options

- **Quinoa Salad with Roasted Vegetables**: Toss cooked quinoa with roasted sweet potatoes, zucchini, and bell peppers. Add a handful of spinach and a sprinkle of pumpkin seeds for crunch. Quinoa is a complete protein and helps reduce inflammation, while the colorful vegetables provide antioxidants.
- **Grilled Chicken with Spinach and Avocado Salad**: Marinate chicken in olive oil, lemon, and garlic, then grill. Serve it over a bed of spinach, avocado, and cherry tomatoes. Olive oil and avocado are rich in monounsaturated fats, which help lower inflammation.

Snack Ideas

- **Hummus and Veggie Sticks**: Enjoy a handful of crunchy veggies like cucumber, carrots, and celery with a serving of homemade or store-bought hummus. Hummus provides plant-based protein and healthy fats.
- **Mixed Nuts and Dark Chocolate**: A small handful of almonds, walnuts, and a few squares of dark chocolate (at least 70% cacao) can curb cravings while providing antioxidants and healthy fats.

Dinner Options

- **Salmon with Steamed Broccoli and Brown Rice**: Grill or bake a fillet of wild-caught salmon and serve it with steamed broccoli and a side of brown rice. Salmon is high in omega-3 fatty acids, which are excellent for reducing inflammation and lowering cortisol.
- **Lentil Stew with Turmeric and Ginger**: Cook lentils with diced tomatoes, garlic, turmeric, and ginger. Serve this hearty stew with a side of roasted cauliflower for an anti-inflammatory punch.

Hydration and Beverages

- **Green Tea**: Replace sugary drinks and coffee with green tea, which contains antioxidants that help reduce inflammation and lower cortisol. The amino acid **L-theanine** in green tea promotes calm and focused energy without the jittery side effects of caffeine.
- **Infused Water**: Add slices of cucumber, mint, or lemon to your water for extra flavor and a gentle detox effect that supports hydration and overall stress relief.

This meal plan is designed to be easy to follow and flexible, so feel free to mix and match meals based on your preferences. The anti-inflammatory ingredients in these recipes will help you lower cortisol levels, promote better energy, and set the stage for long-term wellness.

Daily Routines to Boost Energy

During the first week of your reset, incorporating simple daily routines can have a significant impact on your energy levels and overall well-being. By building habits that support natural energy production and reduce stress, you can help your body recharge and feel more balanced throughout the day. These routines are designed to align with your body's natural rhythms, support cortisol regulation, and give you the stamina needed to navigate daily tasks with ease.

1. Morning Sunlight Exposure

Getting exposure to natural sunlight early in the day is one of the most effective ways to regulate your circadian rhythm and boost energy. Sunlight signals to your body that it's time to wake up, helps regulate cortisol levels, and improves mood by increasing serotonin production.

- **How to incorporate it**: Spend 10-15 minutes outside in the morning, even if it's just standing by a sunny window or going for a short walk. This practice helps set the tone for the day by reducing morning grogginess and increasing alertness.
- **Why it works**: Sunlight exposure regulates your body's internal clock, which helps balance cortisol and improves energy throughout the day.

2. Hydration First Thing in the Morning

After hours of sleep, your body is naturally dehydrated, and this can contribute to feelings of fatigue. Rehydrating first thing in the morning helps kickstart your metabolism and boosts energy levels.

- **How to incorporate it**: Before breakfast or coffee, drink a large glass of water with a squeeze of lemon. The lemon adds a dose of vitamin C, which supports adrenal health and detoxification.
- **Why it works**: Proper hydration helps improve cognitive function, maintain energy, and reduce the stress response that dehydration can trigger.

3. Morning Movement

Starting your day with light physical activity can help boost your energy and mood, enhance blood flow, and reduce morning cortisol levels. The key is choosing gentle, low-stress exercises that invigorate your body without causing fatigue.

- **How to incorporate it**: Incorporate a short 10-15 minute routine that includes stretches, yoga, or a brisk walk. Focus on gentle movements that energize the body and reduce stiffness.
- **Why it works**: Movement increases blood circulation and promotes the release of endorphins, which reduce stress and improve mood. Gentle morning exercise can also help regulate your body's cortisol levels, making you feel more balanced throughout the day.

4. Midday Mindfulness Break

As the day progresses, stress levels can rise, which can lead to an energy slump in the afternoon. Taking a brief mindfulness break in the middle of the day helps reduce stress, improve focus, and recharge your energy levels.

- **How to incorporate it**: Set aside 5-10 minutes for mindfulness practice, such as deep breathing, meditation, or simply stepping away from your desk for a mental reset. Use this time to focus on your breath or take a short walk outside.
- **Why it works**: Mindfulness practices reduce cortisol production by calming the nervous system and improving mental clarity, making you feel more refreshed and energized.

5. Balanced, Energy-Boosting Snacks

What you eat during the day can have a major impact on your energy levels. Choosing the right snacks will help maintain stable blood sugar and prevent the dreaded afternoon energy crash that often follows sugary or processed snacks.

- **How to incorporate it**: Opt for snacks that combine protein, healthy fats, and fiber, such as a handful of nuts with an apple, hummus with carrot sticks, or Greek yogurt with chia seeds.
- **Why it works**: These balanced snacks provide sustained energy, stabilize blood sugar, and prevent the spikes and crashes that can lead to low energy and high cortisol.

6. Consistent Bedtime Routine

Restorative sleep is essential for managing stress and boosting energy. A consistent bedtime routine helps prepare your body for sleep by signaling that it's time to wind down. This routine should prioritize relaxation and support the natural reduction of cortisol before bed.

- **How to incorporate it**: Create a pre-bed routine that involves dimming lights, avoiding screens, and engaging in calming activities like reading or light stretching. Aim to go to bed at the same time each night.
- **Why it works**: Consistency in your sleep routine helps regulate your circadian rhythm, promotes better sleep quality, and ensures you wake up feeling more refreshed and energized.

By incorporating these simple routines into your daily life, you can create a strong foundation for energy management, stress reduction, and cortisol regulation. Each habit works synergistically to help your body reset, recharge, and stay balanced throughout the day.

CHAPTER 17

Week 2 – Balance and Energize

Adding Gut-Healing Foods to Your Diet

In Week 2 of your reset, the focus shifts toward healing and balancing your gut. The gut is closely linked to how your body manages stress and regulates cortisol levels. By incorporating gut-healing foods into your diet, you can not only improve digestion but also support a healthier stress response and enhance your energy levels. A well-functioning gut leads to better nutrient absorption, reduced inflammation, and balanced hormones, all of which contribute to a more energized, balanced you.

Why Gut Health Matters for Stress Management

Your gut microbiome—the community of microorganisms living in your digestive system—plays a critical role in your overall health, including how your body responds to stress. An imbalanced gut can lead to increased inflammation, which can trigger higher cortisol levels, fatigue, and mood swings. Additionally, the gut communicates directly with the brain through the gut-brain axis, influencing your mental and emotional well-being.

- **Gut and cortisol regulation**: A healthy gut supports the regulation of cortisol, ensuring that stress hormones are kept in check. This helps you feel calmer and more in control during stressful situations.

- **Gut and energy**: When your gut is functioning properly, your body absorbs more nutrients from food, helping you feel more energized throughout the day.

Key Gut-Healing Foods to Include

Here are some of the most effective gut-healing foods to add to your diet this week. These foods will help repair your gut lining, promote the growth of beneficial bacteria, and reduce inflammation.

1. Fermented Foods

Fermented foods are rich in probiotics—beneficial bacteria that support a healthy gut microbiome. These bacteria help balance the digestive system by promoting the growth of good bacteria and inhibiting harmful bacteria. They also play a role in reducing inflammation, which is essential for managing cortisol levels.

- **Examples**: Sauerkraut, kimchi, kefir, yogurt (with live cultures), miso, and tempeh.

- **How to incorporate**: Add a spoonful of sauerkraut or kimchi to salads or as a side dish. Include yogurt with live cultures as a snack or breakfast option. Sip on kefir as a refreshing probiotic-rich drink.

2. Bone Broth

Bone broth is an excellent source of collagen, gelatin, and amino acids like glutamine, which help repair the gut lining and reduce intestinal permeability. Known for its gut-soothing properties, bone broth is ideal for healing a damaged gut, often caused by stress, poor diet, or inflammation.

- **Why it's beneficial**: Bone broth strengthens the gut lining, preventing toxins and undigested food particles from leaking into the bloodstream (a condition known as leaky gut), which can trigger inflammation and cortisol spikes.

- **How to incorporate**: Sip on bone broth between meals, or use it as a base for soups and stews.

3. Prebiotic-Rich Foods

Prebiotics are a type of fiber that feeds the beneficial bacteria in your gut, helping them thrive. These fibers pass through the digestive system undigested, providing nourishment for the probiotics in your gut. The combination of prebiotics and probiotics is essential for a healthy microbiome.

- **Examples**: Garlic, onions, leeks, asparagus, bananas (especially slightly underripe), and oats.

- **How to incorporate**: Add garlic and onions to your cooking for flavor and gut support. Enjoy a banana as a snack or blend it into a smoothie for added fiber. You can also use oats as a base for breakfast with yogurt or kefir.

4. Leafy Greens

Leafy green vegetables like spinach, kale, and arugula are high in fiber and rich in antioxidants that support overall gut health. They provide essential vitamins and minerals that reduce inflammation and help the gut repair itself.

- **Why it's beneficial**: The fiber in leafy greens helps regulate bowel movements and promotes a diverse gut microbiome. Their anti-inflammatory properties help reduce stress on the gut and lower cortisol.

- **How to incorporate**: Add leafy greens to smoothies, salads, or sauté them as a side dish. You can also toss them into soups or stir-fries for an easy nutrient boost.

5. Berries and Other Antioxidant-Rich Fruits

Berries, particularly blueberries, raspberries, and blackberries, are high in antioxidants and fiber, which are vital for maintaining a healthy gut. Antioxidants reduce inflammation and protect the gut lining, while fiber supports digestion and promotes the growth of good bacteria.

- **Why it's beneficial**: The antioxidants in berries help neutralize free radicals, reducing oxidative stress and inflammation in the gut. This, in turn, supports lower cortisol levels and better stress management.

- **How to incorporate**: Add berries to your morning yogurt, chia pudding, or oatmeal. They can also be eaten as a simple snack or blended into a smoothie.

By incorporating these gut-healing foods into your diet this week, you'll be taking important steps toward balancing your cortisol levels, boosting energy, and improving overall health. These foods not only nourish your body but also support your mental and emotional well-being by promoting a healthier, happier gut.

Meal Plan: Recipes to Balance Cortisol and Energy

In Week 2 of your journey, the focus shifts toward maintaining balanced cortisol levels and enhancing your energy through targeted, nourishing meals. The foods you eat directly affect how your body produces and manages cortisol, which is why this week's meal plan includes recipes specifically designed to promote calm energy and reduce stress. These meals are packed with essential nutrients like antioxidants, fiber, healthy fats, and protein—all key to supporting hormone balance and steady energy levels throughout the day.

Key Principles of the Week 2 Meal Plan

This week's meal plan is built around the following principles to help balance cortisol and boost energy:

- **Steady blood sugar**: Maintaining balanced blood sugar levels is crucial for keeping cortisol in check. Each meal combines fiber, healthy fats, and lean proteins to prevent blood sugar spikes and crashes that can increase cortisol production.
- **Anti-inflammatory ingredients**: Inflammation can lead to elevated cortisol and fatigue. This plan incorporates anti-inflammatory foods like fatty fish, leafy greens, berries, and spices like turmeric and ginger to reduce inflammation and support overall well-being.
- **Gut health support**: Since gut health and cortisol are closely linked, this plan also includes gut-friendly foods like fermented vegetables, bone broth, and fiber-rich fruits and vegetables.

Sample Meal Plan for Balancing Cortisol and Energy

This sample meal plan offers easy-to-follow recipes that balance energy, reduce stress, and keep cortisol in check. Feel free to adjust the meals based on your preferences and lifestyle.

Breakfast Options

- **Overnight Oats with Chia Seeds and Berries**: Combine rolled oats, chia seeds, almond milk, and a handful of fresh berries in a jar. Let it sit overnight, and enjoy a fiber-rich breakfast that supports gut health and provides sustained energy. The chia seeds add omega-3s, while the berries offer antioxidants to help fight inflammation.
- **Green Smoothie with Spinach and Avocado**: Blend spinach, avocado, a banana, and unsweetened almond milk for a creamy, nutrient-packed smoothie. Spinach is rich in magnesium, which helps lower cortisol, while avocado provides healthy fats for energy.

Lunch Options

- **Quinoa Salad with Grilled Salmon and Leafy Greens**: Toss cooked quinoa with arugula, spinach, and grilled salmon. Add a drizzle of olive oil and lemon juice. Quinoa offers fiber and protein to maintain stable blood sugar, while salmon provides anti-inflammatory omega-3 fatty acids to support hormone balance.
- **Lentil and Vegetable Stew**: Simmer lentils with diced carrots, celery, and onions in a rich vegetable broth seasoned with turmeric and garlic. This hearty stew is packed with fiber and plant-based protein to support gut health and cortisol regulation.

Snack Ideas

- **Greek Yogurt with Walnuts and Honey**: A small bowl of unsweetened Greek yogurt topped with walnuts and a drizzle of honey makes for a quick, gut-friendly snack. Yogurt's probiotics support digestion, while walnuts provide omega-3s to lower inflammation.

- **Apple Slices with Almond Butter**: For a quick energy boost, pair apple slices with almond butter. The fiber from the apple and healthy fats from the almond butter help stabilize blood sugar, keeping energy levels steady.

Dinner Options

- **Roasted Chicken with Sweet Potatoes and Steamed Broccoli**: Marinate chicken with olive oil, garlic, and thyme, then roast it alongside cubed sweet potatoes. Serve with steamed broccoli. Sweet potatoes are high in fiber and antioxidants, promoting healthy cortisol levels, while broccoli is rich in vitamins that support adrenal function.
- **Stir-Fried Tofu with Bok Choy and Ginger**: Stir-fry tofu with bok choy, ginger, and sesame oil. Ginger's anti-inflammatory properties help reduce cortisol, while bok choy provides fiber and vitamins that support gut health.

Hydration and Beverages

- **Lemon Water with Mint**: Start your day with a glass of warm lemon water infused with fresh mint. The vitamin C from the lemon supports adrenal health, while mint aids digestion.
- **Herbal Teas**: Throughout the day, sip on calming herbal teas like chamomile or peppermint. These teas have been shown to reduce stress and promote relaxation, helping to keep cortisol levels in check.

By following this meal plan, you're not only providing your body with essential nutrients but also actively working to balance cortisol and enhance your energy levels. These meals are designed to reduce inflammation, support gut health, and provide steady energy, ensuring you feel balanced and energized throughout Week 2.

Introducing Adaptogens for Stress Management

Adaptogens are powerful, natural herbs that have been used for centuries to help the body manage stress and maintain balance. Unlike many supplements that provide temporary relief, adaptogens work by enhancing your body's ability to cope with stress in a sustainable way. They support adrenal function, regulate cortisol levels, and promote resilience to both physical and mental stressors. Incorporating adaptogens into your routine during Week 2 is a powerful step toward balancing cortisol and boosting energy.

What Are Adaptogens?

Adaptogens are a unique class of herbs that help the body adapt to stress. They don't target a single part of the body but rather work holistically, strengthening various systems to create balance. When faced with stress, adaptogens help regulate the production of cortisol, preventing it from spiking too high or dropping too low. This balanced response reduces the harmful effects of chronic stress, such as fatigue, anxiety, and weight gain.

- **How adaptogens work**: By modulating the hypothalamic-pituitary-adrenal (HPA) axis, adaptogens help normalize the body's stress response. Whether your cortisol levels are too high due to stress or too low due to burnout, adaptogens work to restore balance.

Key Adaptogens to Incorporate for Stress Management

Here are three highly effective adaptogens that can be introduced during Week 2 to support stress management and cortisol regulation. Each adaptogen has unique properties, allowing you to choose the ones that best suit your needs.

1. Ashwagandha

Ashwagandha is one of the most well-known adaptogens for reducing cortisol and managing stress. It has been used in Ayurvedic medicine for centuries to calm the nervous system, promote restful sleep, and increase energy.

- **Benefits**: Ashwagandha helps reduce cortisol levels, improving both mental clarity and emotional well-being. It's particularly effective for people who experience anxiety, irritability, or sleep disturbances due to chronic stress.
- **How to incorporate**: You can take ashwagandha as a supplement in capsule or powder form. If you prefer, you can mix the powder into smoothies or herbal teas for easy consumption.

2. Rhodiola Rosea

Rhodiola is known for its ability to enhance physical and mental endurance, making it an excellent choice if you're feeling drained by stress. This adaptogen helps reduce cortisol levels while boosting energy and focus.

- **Benefits**: Rhodiola supports adrenal function and helps prevent burnout. It's especially beneficial for people who experience fatigue, brain fog, or low energy due to stress. It's also known to improve resilience, helping you better manage stress over time.
- **How to incorporate**: Rhodiola is often available in capsule or tincture form. It's best taken earlier in the day because of its energizing effects.

3. Holy Basil (Tulsi)

Holy basil, or tulsi, is revered in Ayurvedic medicine for its calming effects on the mind and body. It's a powerful adaptogen for managing emotional stress, promoting mental clarity, and supporting adrenal health.

- **Benefits**: Holy basil helps lower cortisol levels and reduces inflammation caused by stress. It's also effective at promoting a sense of calm and improving focus, making it great for emotional and mental well-being.
- **How to incorporate**: Holy basil is commonly consumed as a tea. You can enjoy a cup of tulsi tea in the afternoon or evening to help calm the mind and reduce cortisol naturally.

How to Add Adaptogens to Your Daily Routine

Incorporating adaptogens into your routine is simple, and their flexibility allows you to find what works best for your lifestyle. Here are some tips for including them in your daily habits:

- **Start slow**: Begin with a small dose to see how your body responds to each adaptogen. Many adaptogens come in capsules, powders, or tinctures, giving you plenty of options.
- **Consistency is key**: Adaptogens work best when taken consistently over time. Integrate them into your daily routine, whether in your morning smoothie, as an afternoon tea, or in a supplement form with meals.
- **Personalize your regimen**: Choose one or two adaptogens to start with, and tailor them to your specific needs. For example, ashwagandha is great for evening relaxation, while rhodiola may be better in the morning to support energy and focus.

Building Long-Term Resilience

Using adaptogens regularly can help you build long-term resilience to stress, balance your energy, and improve overall well-being. As you introduce adaptogens into your routine this week, focus on the ones that align with your stress-management goals and energy needs. Over time, you'll find that these powerful herbs offer a sustainable way to manage stress, balance cortisol, and enhance your vitality.

CHAPTER 18

Week 3 – Restore and Strengthen

Focusing on Gut Health and Sleep Improvement

In Week 3 of your journey, the focus shifts to two foundational pillars of well-being: gut health and sleep. Both play a crucial role in regulating cortisol, reducing stress, and ensuring your body is able to recover and restore itself. By improving your gut health and sleep patterns, you'll not only enhance your energy levels but also strengthen your resilience to stress. These elements work synergistically—when your gut is healthy, your sleep improves, and when you sleep well, your gut health is supported. This week, we dive into practical strategies to restore both.

Why Gut Health Is Key to Restoring Balance

Your gut is often referred to as the body's "second brain" because of its direct communication with your central nervous system via the gut-brain axis. A healthy gut is essential for stress management because it helps regulate inflammation, supports nutrient absorption, and even influences your mood through serotonin production.

- **Inflammation and cortisol**: Chronic inflammation in the gut can lead to elevated cortisol levels. Gut-friendly foods, such as those rich in prebiotics and probiotics, can help reduce this inflammation, leading to lower cortisol production and better stress management.

- **Serotonin production**: A significant portion of serotonin, the "feel-good" neurotransmitter, is produced in the gut. When your gut is balanced and healthy, your serotonin levels are better regulated, which helps to elevate your mood and reduce anxiety.

Key Gut-Health Strategies for Week 3

1. **Increase Prebiotics and Probiotics**: Prebiotics are fibers that feed good bacteria in your gut, while probiotics are live beneficial bacteria that help maintain gut balance. Together, they promote a healthy microbiome, which is crucial for lowering inflammation and managing stress.

- **Prebiotic-rich foods:** Onions, garlic, leeks, asparagus, bananas (slightly underripe), and oats.

- **Probiotic-rich foods:** Fermented foods like yogurt with live cultures, kefir, sauerkraut, kimchi, and kombucha. Aim to include one or two servings of fermented foods daily to support gut health.

2. **Eat Fiber-Rich Meals**: Fiber promotes regular digestion, reduces inflammation, and supports a healthy gut lining. Consuming fiber-rich meals, particularly those with vegetables, fruits, and whole grains, helps to balance cortisol levels by preventing blood sugar spikes and supporting gut health.

3. **Avoid Processed Foods**: Processed foods, refined sugars, and trans fats contribute to gut in-

flammation and dysbiosis (an imbalance in the gut bacteria). During Week 3, focus on whole, nutrient-dense foods to repair and strengthen your gut.

Improving Sleep for Stress Recovery

Quality sleep is critical for stress management, cortisol regulation, and overall recovery. When you don't get enough sleep, or if your sleep is disrupted, cortisol levels can spike, leading to feelings of anxiety, irritability, and fatigue. This week focuses on optimizing your sleep routine to ensure restorative rest.

1. **Establish a Consistent Sleep Schedule**: One of the most effective ways to improve sleep is to go to bed and wake up at the same time every day, even on weekends. A consistent routine helps regulate your circadian rhythm, which in turn helps balance cortisol levels.
2. **Create a Pre-Bedtime Routine**: Incorporating calming activities into your evening routine can signal to your body that it's time to wind down. Dim the lights an hour before bed, avoid screens, and try activities like reading, light stretching, or meditation.
3. **Optimize Your Sleep Environment**: A comfortable, relaxing environment is key to quality sleep. Make sure your bedroom is cool, dark, and quiet. Using blackout curtains, earplugs, or a white noise machine can help create an optimal sleep environment. Additionally, avoid consuming caffeine or heavy meals close to bedtime.
4. **Consider Natural Sleep Aids**: If stress or anxiety is disrupting your sleep, consider incorporating natural sleep aids like magnesium or herbal teas. Magnesium promotes muscle relaxation and is known to improve sleep quality, while teas like chamomile and valerian root can help calm the nervous system.

How Gut Health and Sleep Work Together

The connection between your gut and sleep is profound. Poor sleep can disrupt the balance of your gut microbiome, leading to digestive issues and heightened cortisol. Conversely, an unhealthy gut can lead to sleep disturbances due to increased inflammation and stress. By focusing on both areas this week, you'll create a positive feedback loop—improving one will naturally enhance the other.

As you implement these strategies in Week 3, you'll notice improved energy, better digestion, and a greater ability to manage stress. Prioritizing gut health and sleep is key to feeling restored, strong, and ready to take on the next phase of your wellness journey.

Meal Plan: Nutrient-Dense Meals for Recovery

In Week 3, the focus is on providing your body with nutrient-dense meals that promote recovery, strengthen your immune system, and enhance your ability to manage stress. These meals are designed to replenish your energy stores, repair tissues, and support optimal cortisol regulation. By prioritizing whole, unprocessed foods rich in essential vitamins, minerals, and healthy fats, this plan will help your body restore balance and resilience.

Key Principles for Nutrient-Dense Meals

- **Anti-inflammatory ingredients**: Inflammation can exacerbate stress and hinder recovery. This meal plan emphasizes anti-inflammatory foods like leafy greens, omega-3 rich fish, and spices like turmeric and ginger.

- **Protein for repair**: Protein is crucial for tissue repair and maintaining muscle mass, especially when you're working to recover from physical or emotional stress.
- **Healthy fats**: Fats like those found in avocados, nuts, seeds, and olive oil help support brain function, reduce inflammation, and provide sustained energy.
- **Fiber for gut health**: Fiber from whole grains, fruits, and vegetables supports a healthy gut microbiome, which is critical for reducing cortisol and improving digestion.

Sample Nutrient-Dense Meal Plan for Recovery

Here's a sample meal plan for Week 3 that focuses on recovery through nutrient-dense, healing foods. The meals are designed to be simple, delicious, and effective in helping your body recover from stress and replenish energy.

Breakfast Options

- **Sweet Potato and Spinach Scramble**: Sauté cubed sweet potatoes in olive oil until tender, then add a handful of spinach and scramble in two eggs. Sweet potatoes are rich in beta-carotene and fiber, while eggs provide essential amino acids for muscle repair.
- **Chia Pudding with Almond Butter and Berries**: Combine chia seeds, almond milk, and a tablespoon of almond butter in a jar and refrigerate overnight. Top with fresh berries in the morning. Chia seeds are high in omega-3s and fiber, and the berries offer powerful antioxidants to reduce inflammation.

Lunch Options

- **Quinoa Bowl with Grilled Chicken and Avocado**: Cook quinoa and top with grilled chicken, avocado slices, and a drizzle of olive oil. Add some leafy greens like kale or arugula for an extra nutrient boost. Quinoa is a complete protein, and avocados provide healthy fats that support brain health and hormone balance.
- **Lentil Soup with Carrots and Turmeric**: Simmer lentils with chopped carrots, onions, garlic, and turmeric for a hearty, anti-inflammatory meal. Lentils are rich in fiber and plant-based protein, while turmeric helps reduce inflammation and supports cortisol balance.

Snack Ideas

- **Mixed Nuts and Dark Chocolate**: A handful of mixed nuts (almonds, walnuts, cashews) with a few squares of dark chocolate (70% cacao or higher) makes for a satisfying, nutrient-dense snack. Nuts provide healthy fats and magnesium, which is key for stress relief.
- **Greek Yogurt with Flaxseeds and Honey**: A small bowl of unsweetened Greek yogurt topped with a tablespoon of flaxseeds and a drizzle of honey provides probiotics for gut health and omega-3s for inflammation reduction.

Dinner Options

- **Baked Salmon with Roasted Vegetables**: Marinate a salmon fillet with olive oil, lemon, and garlic, and bake alongside a mix of vegetables like broccoli, cauliflower, and bell peppers. Salmon is rich in omega-3s, which reduce inflammation and support adrenal health, while the vegetables provide fiber and antioxidants for gut health.

- **Stir-Fried Tofu with Bok Choy and Ginger**: Stir-fry tofu in sesame oil with bok choy, garlic, and ginger. Ginger's anti-inflammatory properties help reduce cortisol, and tofu provides plant-based protein to support recovery.

Hydration and Beverages

- **Green Tea**: Sip on green tea throughout the day. It contains antioxidants and the amino acid L-theanine, which helps promote relaxation and focus without increasing cortisol.
- **Cucumber and Mint-Infused Water**: Staying hydrated is essential for recovery. Adding slices of cucumber and mint to your water can provide a refreshing, mild detox effect while supporting digestion.

This nutrient-dense meal plan focuses on providing your body with everything it needs to recover from stress, reduce inflammation, and restore energy levels. These meals are rich in essential nutrients, ensuring you feel stronger, more energized, and better equipped to handle the demands of everyday life.

Daily Movement and Stress Management Tips

In Week 3, you'll focus on incorporating gentle, restorative movement and stress management techniques to strengthen your body and enhance your mental well-being. Movement is essential for reducing cortisol, promoting relaxation, and boosting your energy levels, while stress management helps you build resilience and balance your emotions. This week's focus is on sustainable practices that help you restore and recharge, without overwhelming your body or mind.

Importance of Movement for Cortisol Regulation

Movement plays a critical role in balancing cortisol levels. Gentle, restorative exercises, such as walking, yoga, and stretching, reduce cortisol by encouraging blood flow, releasing tension, and promoting the production of endorphins—your body's natural mood elevators. Unlike intense exercise, which can spike cortisol if done excessively, these types of movements help you maintain a balanced stress response without overburdening your adrenal system.

Suggested Daily Movement Practices

1. **Morning Stretching Routine**: Start your day with a 5-10 minute stretching routine to wake up your muscles, improve circulation, and set a positive tone for the day. Focus on gentle stretches that lengthen the spine, open the chest, and relax the neck and shoulders. This routine helps reduce morning stiffness and releases any tension that may have built up overnight.
- *Example moves:* Cat-cow stretches, forward folds, and neck rolls.
- Why **it works:** Gentle morning movement activates the parasympathetic nervous system, reducing cortisol and helping you feel more energized and relaxed throughout the day.
2. **Walking or Light Cardio**: Incorporating a daily walk, whether it's during your lunch break or after dinner, is an excellent way to lower cortisol and boost energy. Aim for 20-30 minutes of walking, and try to get outdoors if possible for added benefits of sunlight and fresh air.

- **Why it works:** Walking at a moderate pace helps regulate cortisol, clears your mind, and supports overall cardiovascular health without putting stress on your body.

3. **Evening Yoga or Gentle Pilates**: Yoga and Pilates are both fantastic ways to wind down in the evening. These practices focus on controlled, mindful movements that build core strength, improve flexibility, and encourage deep, calming breathing. Consider a 15-20 minute session that includes gentle stretches, deep breathing, and restorative poses like child's pose or legs-up-the-wall.

- **Why it works:** Evening movement helps lower cortisol levels and prepares your body for restful sleep by releasing physical tension and calming your nervous system.

Stress Management Techniques for Week 3

Stress management is just as important as physical movement in this phase of your recovery. Incorporating daily stress-reducing practices helps to lower cortisol, improve focus, and prevent emotional burnout.

1. **Deep Breathing Exercises**: Take 5-10 minutes each day to practice deep breathing. Focus on slow, controlled breaths, inhaling through your nose for four counts, holding for four counts, and exhaling slowly through your mouth for four counts. This simple practice can immediately calm your nervous system and lower cortisol levels.

- **Why it works:** Deep breathing stimulates the parasympathetic nervous system, signaling to your body that it's safe to relax and reduce cortisol.

2. **Mindful Meditation**: Set aside a few minutes each day for mindful meditation. Whether it's in the morning, during a break, or before bed, mindfulness helps bring awareness to the present moment, easing stress and preventing your mind from wandering into worry or overthinking.

- **How to practice:** Sit comfortably in a quiet space, close your eyes, and focus on your breath. If your mind starts to wander, gently bring your focus back to your breath without judgment.

- **Why it works:** Regular mindfulness practice has been shown to lower cortisol and improve emotional regulation, making it easier to manage stress throughout the day.

3. **Gratitude Journaling**: Writing down three things you're grateful for each day is a simple yet powerful way to shift your mindset away from stress and negativity. This practice can be done in the morning to set a positive tone for the day or in the evening to reflect on the day's highlights.

- **Why it works:** Focusing on gratitude reduces cortisol and enhances feelings of well-being by encouraging positive thinking and reducing the mental load of stress.

Building Consistency in Movement and Stress Management

The key to success in Week 3 is consistency. These practices are designed to be sustainable and easily incorporated into your daily routine. By adding gentle movement and stress management techniques to your day, you'll improve your cortisol balance, boost your energy, and build long-term resilience to stress. Make sure to listen to your body and adjust your routine as needed—rest and recovery are just as important as movement in maintaining a healthy stress response.

CHAPTER 19

Week 4 – Sustain and Thrive

Maintaining Results with Balanced Eating and Stress Relief

As you enter Week 4, your focus shifts toward maintaining the progress you've made. By now, you've reset your body, balanced your cortisol levels, and learned to manage stress more effectively. This final week emphasizes sustaining these results through balanced eating and ongoing stress relief strategies. The goal is to create habits that not only keep your cortisol levels in check but also promote long-term vitality, helping you thrive in daily life.

Balanced Eating for Sustained Cortisol Control

Balanced eating is key to maintaining the improvements you've made. The foods you consume play a significant role in keeping cortisol levels low, regulating blood sugar, and supporting overall energy. Here are the core principles of balanced eating that will help you stay on track:

- **Focus on whole, unprocessed foods**: Continue to prioritize whole, nutrient-dense foods such as vegetables, fruits, lean proteins, and healthy fats. These foods provide the vitamins and minerals your body needs to support adrenal health, reduce inflammation, and regulate hormones.
- **Include protein with every meal**: Protein helps stabilize blood sugar, which in turn prevents cortisol spikes. Whether it's plant-based sources like beans and tofu or lean animal proteins like chicken and fish, aim to include a serving of protein with every meal to keep your energy steady throughout the day.
- **Prioritize healthy fats**: Healthy fats, like those found in avocados, olive oil, and fatty fish, are crucial for hormone regulation and brain function. These fats also help curb cravings and keep you feeling satisfied, reducing the chances of overeating and blood sugar fluctuations.
- **Eat regularly, but listen to your body**: Regular, balanced meals help prevent cortisol spikes that come from dips in blood sugar. However, it's equally important to tune into your body's hunger and fullness cues. Avoid stress eating by practicing mindful eating, savoring each bite, and stopping when you feel satisfied rather than full.

Stress Relief Techniques for Ongoing Balance

Maintaining low cortisol levels also means integrating stress management techniques into your daily life. Stress is inevitable, but how you respond to it can make all the difference in how your body manages cortisol. Incorporating the following stress relief techniques can help you keep cortisol levels in check and prevent the buildup of chronic stress:

- **Practice daily mindfulness or meditation**: Even five minutes of mindfulness or meditation each day can have a profound effect on stress levels. Mindfulness helps bring your awareness to the present moment, reducing anxiety and promoting a sense of calm.

- **Physical movement as stress relief**: Incorporate gentle movement into your routine, such as yoga, walking, or stretching. These activities not only improve physical health but also have a direct impact on lowering cortisol and releasing built-up tension.

- **Prioritize sleep**: Quality sleep is one of the most effective ways to keep cortisol levels balanced. Establish a consistent sleep routine and aim for 7-9 hours of restorative sleep each night. Avoid screens before bed and create a calming bedtime ritual to help you unwind.

- **Set boundaries and prioritize self-care**: Learning to say no to overwhelming demands and prioritizing self-care is essential for long-term stress management. Whether it's taking time for yourself to read, go for a walk, or simply relax, these moments of self-care are necessary to maintain balance.

Building a Long-Term Mindset

As you maintain these habits, it's important to recognize that balance doesn't mean perfection. Life is full of ups and downs, and there will be times when stress levels rise. The key is to develop a flexible mindset where you can adapt, adjust, and return to your habits without guilt or frustration. Sustainable success comes from consistency over time, rather than rigid adherence to rules. Give yourself the grace to manage stress in a way that fits your lifestyle, and remember that each day offers a new opportunity to nourish your body and mind.

By focusing on balanced eating and integrating stress relief practices, you'll be well-equipped to maintain your results and continue thriving. The journey doesn't end here; rather, it's the foundation for a healthier, more resilient life ahead. Keep using the tools you've learned, stay consistent, and enjoy the benefits of a balanced, cortisol-friendly lifestyle.

Meal Plan: Recipes to Keep Cortisol Low

As you move into Week 4, maintaining balanced cortisol levels through nourishing, low-stress meals is key to your long-term success. This week's meal plan focuses on foods that help keep cortisol levels stable while providing the energy you need to thrive. The goal is to integrate simple, nutrient-dense meals that are easy to prepare and sustain you throughout the day, reducing stress on your body and mind.

Key Principles for Cortisol-Lowering Meals

To keep cortisol levels low, your meals should focus on:

- **Stable blood sugar**: Blood sugar fluctuations can trigger cortisol spikes. To avoid this, meals should contain a balance of fiber, protein, and healthy fats, which help slow digestion and maintain steady energy levels.

- **Anti-inflammatory ingredients**: Chronic inflammation raises cortisol levels, so incorporating anti-inflammatory foods is critical. Focus on fresh vegetables, fruits, whole grains, lean proteins, and healthy fats.

- **Magnesium-rich foods**: Magnesium helps regulate cortisol and calm the nervous system. Dark leafy greens, nuts, seeds, and legumes are excellent sources to include in your meals.

Here's a meal plan designed to keep cortisol low, focusing on balance and nutrient density. These recipes are simple yet effective for promoting ongoing cortisol regulation.

Breakfast Options

- **Avocado Toast with Poached Eggs**: Toast a slice of whole-grain bread and top it with half an avocado and two poached eggs. Avocado provides healthy fats that support hormone regulation, while eggs offer protein to keep blood sugar stable.
- **Oatmeal with Berries and Almonds**: Prepare a bowl of steel-cut oats, topping it with fresh berries and a handful of almonds. The fiber from the oats and the antioxidants in the berries help regulate blood sugar, while almonds provide magnesium to lower cortisol.

Lunch Options

- **Grilled Chicken Salad with Spinach and Quinoa**: Toss together grilled chicken, fresh spinach, and cooked quinoa with a lemon-olive oil dressing. Spinach is rich in magnesium, and quinoa provides plant-based protein and fiber, keeping you full and your blood sugar stable.
- **Lentil Soup with Carrots and Kale**: Cook lentils with diced carrots, kale, garlic, and turmeric for an anti-inflammatory, nutrient-dense soup. Lentils are high in fiber and plant-based protein, while turmeric helps reduce inflammation, making this soup perfect for lowering cortisol.

Snack Ideas

- **Greek Yogurt with Flaxseeds**: A small bowl of unsweetened Greek yogurt topped with flaxseeds provides probiotics to support gut health and omega-3s to lower inflammation. These elements help regulate cortisol and maintain energy levels.
- **Apple Slices with Almond Butter**: Slice an apple and enjoy it with a tablespoon of almond butter. Apples are high in fiber, and almond butter provides healthy fats and magnesium to help keep cortisol levels in check.

Dinner Options

- **Baked Salmon with Roasted Sweet Potatoes and Broccoli**: Bake a salmon fillet with olive oil and herbs, and roast sweet potatoes and broccoli on the side. Salmon is rich in omega-3 fatty acids, which reduce inflammation and cortisol, while sweet potatoes provide fiber and vitamins to promote gut health.
- **Stir-Fried Tofu with Brown Rice and Vegetables**: Sauté tofu with garlic, ginger, and mixed vegetables such as bell peppers, broccoli, and snap peas. Serve with brown rice for a fiber-rich, plant-based meal that supports adrenal function and helps keep stress hormones balanced.

Beverages and Hydration

Staying hydrated is essential for cortisol management. Consider these options to complement your meals:

- **Herbal Teas**: Sip on chamomile or peppermint tea to relax your nervous system and lower cortisol naturally.
- **Water with Lemon and Cucumber**: Keep your body hydrated and refreshed with a glass of water infused with lemon slices and cucumber, which helps detoxify and reduce stress.

By following this meal plan, you'll be providing your body with the nutrients it needs to maintain low cortisol levels, stabilize blood sugar, and support a calm, focused mind. These meals are designed to be balanced, easy to prepare, and effective for keeping you on track with your long-term health goals.

Long-Term Strategies to Avoid Burnout

As you enter the final week of your program, it's crucial to establish long-term strategies to prevent burnout and ensure sustained health and well-being. Burnout occurs when stress becomes chronic, overwhelming your body's ability to recover. Over time, this can lead to fatigue, mood swings, and increased cortisol levels, undoing the progress you've made. By incorporating the following long-term strategies into your daily routine, you can stay balanced, maintain low cortisol levels, and avoid the trap of burnout.

Prioritize Rest and Recovery

One of the most effective ways to prevent burnout is to prioritize rest and recovery as part of your regular routine. It's easy to feel the pressure to constantly be productive, but adequate rest is essential for maintaining your energy and emotional balance.

- **Make sleep a non-negotiable**: Aim for 7-9 hours of sleep each night. Develop a consistent bedtime routine that signals to your body that it's time to wind down, such as dimming the lights, avoiding screens, and practicing relaxation techniques like deep breathing or meditation.
- **Schedule regular downtime**: Build regular breaks into your day, even if they're just 5-10 minutes of quiet time to step away from work or obligations. These mini-breaks allow you to reset mentally and physically, preventing stress from accumulating.

Set Boundaries to Protect Your Energy

Burnout often stems from taking on too much and not setting boundaries. Learning to say no and setting clear limits around your time and energy can protect you from becoming overwhelmed. These boundaries apply to both work and personal obligations.

- **Learn to say no**: Saying no to unnecessary commitments or obligations that drain your energy is essential for maintaining balance. Practice setting limits with kindness and clarity, focusing on what aligns with your priorities and well-being.
- **Balance work and life**: It's important to maintain a clear separation between work time and personal time. Set boundaries around when you're available for work tasks and ensure you're dedicating enough time to self-care and leisure activities.

Incorporate Regular Movement and Stress-Relieving Activities

Incorporating regular physical activity into your routine is one of the best ways to keep stress at bay. Movement doesn't need to be intense to be effective—gentle, restorative exercises are excellent for lowering cortisol and preventing burnout.

- **Gentle daily movement**: Incorporate walking, yoga, or stretching into your daily routine. These activities are easy to maintain and offer significant mental and physical benefits, including reduced stress and improved mood.
- **Mindful movement**: Try exercises that combine movement and mindfulness, such as tai chi or Pilates. These practices help you stay present while promoting relaxation and flexibility.

Practice Self-Compassion and Mindfulness

A key part of avoiding burnout is shifting your mindset toward self-compassion. Being kind to yourself during challenging times, rather than critical or self-demanding, can make a huge difference in your stress levels.

- **Develop a mindfulness practice**: Mindfulness teaches you to focus on the present moment rather than dwelling on the past or worrying about the future. Even a few minutes a day of mindful breathing or meditation can significantly lower cortisol and reduce the risk of burnout.
- **Celebrate small wins**: Acknowledge your progress, no matter how small. Celebrating the little achievements helps build momentum and prevents you from feeling overwhelmed by bigger tasks.

Nourish Your Body with Regular, Balanced Meals

Long-term energy and cortisol management depend on consistent, balanced nutrition. Skipping meals or eating processed foods regularly can contribute to imbalanced blood sugar, which spikes cortisol and leaves you feeling depleted.

- **Eat regularly**: Avoid skipping meals by planning ahead and keeping healthy snacks available. Eating at regular intervals helps prevent energy crashes and keeps cortisol levels stable.
- **Focus on whole foods**: Continue to prioritize meals rich in whole foods, such as vegetables, lean proteins, healthy fats, and complex carbohydrates. These foods provide sustained energy and reduce the risk of blood sugar spikes, which can trigger cortisol release.

Build a Support Network

No one can do it all alone. Building a supportive community around you—whether through friends, family, or professional relationships—helps reduce feelings of isolation and provides a buffer against stress.

- **Reach out for support**: If you're feeling overwhelmed, don't hesitate to ask for help. Whether it's delegating tasks at work or talking to a trusted friend, having a support system can prevent burnout from creeping in.
- **Connect regularly**: Stay connected with loved ones, even if it's just a quick chat or coffee break. Social connections reduce stress and give you a sense of belonging and security.

By integrating these strategies into your daily life, you'll create a foundation of balance and resilience that prevents burnout and allows you to thrive long-term. Keep focusing on what nourishes both your body and mind, and remember that preventing burnout is about taking small, consistent steps to protect your energy and well-being.

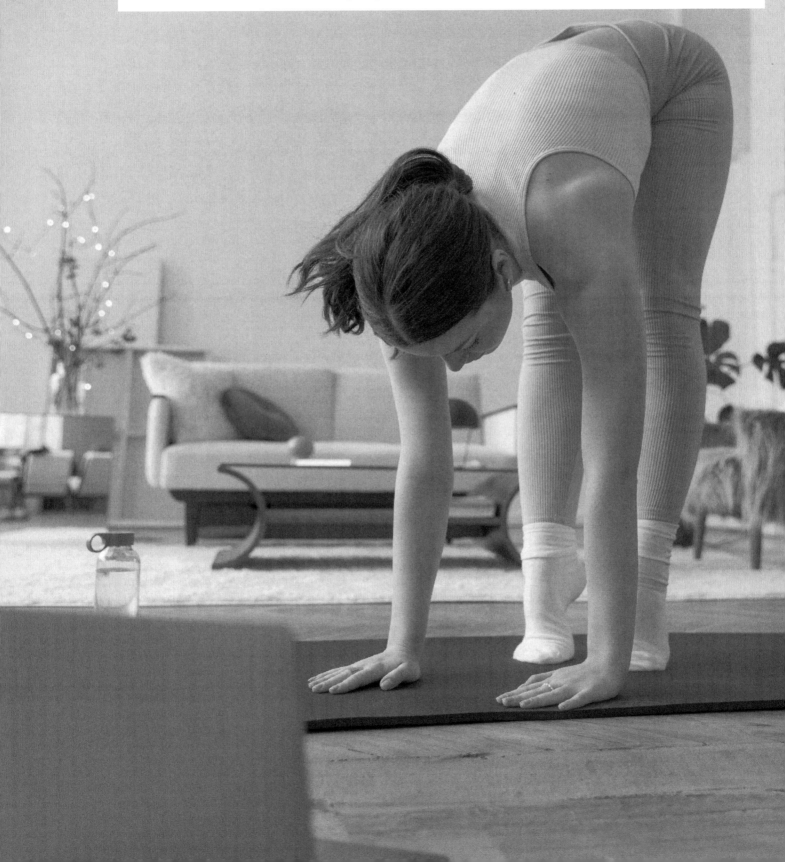

Achieving Long-Term Success

Making the 7 Pillars Part of Your Daily Life

How to Maintain Cortisol Balance for the Long Term

Maintaining balanced cortisol levels for the long term is about integrating sustainable habits into your daily life. After completing the initial detox and reset phases, the challenge becomes keeping cortisol in check without returning to old patterns of stress and imbalance. The key to long-term success is adopting a flexible approach, recognizing that life will have its ups and downs, but with the right tools, you can keep your stress response under control and thrive.

Prioritize Consistent, Balanced Eating

One of the most effective ways to maintain cortisol balance is by sticking to a nutrient-dense, whole foods-based diet that supports stable blood sugar levels. Avoid letting stress push you into skipping meals or resorting to processed foods, which can cause blood sugar spikes and, in turn, trigger cortisol.

- **Maintain regular meal times**: Eating at consistent intervals throughout the day prevents the blood sugar crashes that can elevate cortisol. Aim for three meals and two snacks that include a balance of lean proteins, healthy fats, and complex carbohydrates.

- **Hydrate adequately**: Dehydration is a common trigger for cortisol spikes. Ensure you're drinking enough water throughout the day, especially if you're physically active or live in a dry climate.

- **Continue incorporating anti-inflammatory foods**: Foods like leafy greens, berries, fatty fish, and olive oil not only nourish your body but help combat inflammation, keeping cortisol in check. Make these a regular part of your meals.

Move Your Body—But Keep It Gentle

Regular movement is essential for long-term cortisol regulation, but it's important to strike the right balance between exertion and recovery. While high-intensity workouts have their place, gentle, restorative movement should be a part of your daily routine to avoid stressing your adrenal system.

- **Daily low-impact activities**: Incorporate walking, yoga, or stretching into your day. These activities help calm your nervous system, promote circulation, and support overall hormonal balance without overtaxing your body.

- **Restorative exercise routines**: Engage in activities like Pilates or swimming that are gentle on your joints and muscles while still offering physical benefits. These types of exercises reduce cortisol without the risk of overstimulation.

Prioritize Sleep as a Non-Negotiable

Sleep is one of the most powerful tools for regulating cortisol. When you're sleep-deprived, your body compensates by raising cortisol levels, which leads to fatigue, cravings, and emotional instability.

- **Stick to a consistent sleep schedule**: Go to bed and wake up at the same time each day, even on weekends. A consistent routine helps regulate your circadian rhythm and keeps cortisol levels steady.
- **Create a sleep-friendly environment**: Ensure your bedroom is conducive to sleep—cool, dark, and quiet. Invest in blackout curtains, white noise machines, or anything else that helps you wind down.

Manage Emotional Stress

Emotional stress is one of the most significant contributors to elevated cortisol. Managing your emotional well-being through mindfulness practices and stress reduction techniques will help you stay balanced even in challenging situations.

- **Practice mindfulness or meditation**: Taking just 5-10 minutes a day for mindfulness or meditation can help reduce anxiety and calm your nervous system, keeping cortisol levels from rising. Focus on deep breathing and letting go of stressors from the day.
- **Set boundaries and protect your energy**: One of the best ways to manage stress is by learning to say no and setting clear boundaries with work, family, or social obligations. Protecting your energy is essential to avoid burnout and keep cortisol levels in check.

Build Resilience through Self-Care

Long-term cortisol balance requires a holistic approach to self-care. The more you nurture your mental, emotional, and physical health, the better your body can cope with life's inevitable stressors.

- **Incorporate daily self-care rituals**: Whether it's a morning routine that involves stretching and deep breathing or an evening bath with essential oils, build self-care into your daily life. These moments of care help calm your nervous system and keep cortisol levels balanced.
- **Find joy and connection**: Regularly engage in activities that bring you joy and help you feel connected to others. Laughter, meaningful conversations, and creative hobbies all support a healthy mindset and help reduce cortisol production.

Regular Check-ins and Adjustments

Maintaining cortisol balance for the long term requires self-awareness and regular check-ins with yourself. Be mindful of how your body responds to stress and adjust your habits as needed. If you notice signs of heightened cortisol—such as trouble sleeping, increased cravings, or feeling anxious—revisit the tools that have worked for you during the reset process.

By consistently applying these long-term strategies, you'll keep cortisol levels in check, build resilience, and create a life where stress doesn't control you. Balance is not about being perfect, but about maintaining the tools to thrive and feel your best every day.

Time-Saving Tips to Stay on Track

Staying consistent with your cortisol-balancing routine doesn't have to be time-consuming or overwhelming. By integrating smart, time-saving strategies, you can maintain your results with minimal effort, making it easier to stick with the habits that support your health and well-being. These tips are designed for busy women who want to prioritize their health while balancing the demands of work, family, and daily life.

Plan and Prep Your Meals Ahead of Time

Meal prepping is one of the most effective ways to save time while staying on track with balanced, cortisol-friendly eating. By planning and preparing meals in advance, you'll eliminate the stress of last-minute food decisions, avoid unhealthy choices, and ensure you have nourishing meals ready to go throughout the week.

- **Batch cooking**: Set aside one day each week, such as Sunday, to batch cook meals for the next few days. Focus on simple, versatile recipes like soups, stir-fries, or roasted vegetables and proteins that can be easily reheated or mixed into different meals.
- **Pre-chop ingredients**: Save time during the week by pre-chopping vegetables, portioning out snacks, and preparing components for meals like grains, proteins, or salads. Store them in airtight containers for easy assembly when it's time to eat.
- **Use slow cookers or instant pots**: Invest in time-saving kitchen tools like a slow cooker or Instant Pot, which allow you to prepare meals with minimal hands-on effort. These appliances can cook meals while you're busy, freeing up time for other tasks.

Streamline Your Exercise Routine

Staying active is crucial for cortisol balance, but finding time for exercise can feel challenging. By optimizing your movement routine, you can still get the benefits of physical activity without spending hours at the gym.

- **Focus on short, effective workouts**: Rather than spending an hour or more on exercise, aim for 20-30 minute sessions that combine cardio and strength training. High-intensity interval training (HIIT) or circuit workouts are great for boosting energy, lowering cortisol, and saving time.
- **Incorporate movement into your daily routine**: Look for opportunities to add gentle movement throughout your day. Take short walks during breaks, stretch at your desk, or do bodyweight exercises while watching TV. These small bursts of activity can add up without taking a large chunk out of your day.
- **Set a consistent schedule**: Having a regular time slot for movement can make it easier to stay on track. Whether it's a morning yoga session or an afternoon walk, scheduling your workouts in advance ensures you prioritize exercise without it feeling like a burden.

Use Stress Management Techniques on the Go

Stress management doesn't have to be time-intensive. You can incorporate quick, easy stress-relief techniques into your busy day, helping you manage cortisol levels even when you're on the go.

- **Practice deep breathing**: Deep breathing exercises can be done anywhere, anytime, and take only a few minutes. If you feel stressed during the day, pause for a few deep breaths, focusing on slow inhalation and exhalation. This calms your nervous system and helps lower cortisol.

- **Use mindfulness apps**: If you find it difficult to set aside time for meditation or relaxation, use mindfulness apps like Headspace or Calm for guided 5-10 minute sessions that fit into your busy schedule. These short practices can help you de-stress without taking up too much time.
- **Set mini-break reminders**: Use your phone or computer to set reminders for short, 1-2 minute breaks throughout the day. Use this time to stretch, breathe deeply, or take a quick walk, giving your mind and body a chance to reset.

Maximize Your Sleep Routine

Sleep is a powerful tool for maintaining cortisol balance, and optimizing your sleep routine can make a big difference in how rested and energized you feel. A few simple changes can help you get quality sleep without taking up more of your time.

- **Create a calming bedtime ritual**: Wind down with a consistent pre-sleep routine that signals to your body that it's time to rest. This can include a warm bath, reading a book, or practicing relaxation exercises. Even 10-15 minutes of this routine can improve sleep quality.
- **Set a sleep schedule**: Go to bed and wake up at the same time every day, even on weekends. A consistent sleep schedule trains your body to fall asleep faster and wake up more refreshed, helping you manage cortisol levels more effectively.

By incorporating these time-saving strategies, you'll stay on track with your cortisol-balancing lifestyle while freeing up time for the things that matter most. These tips make it easier to integrate healthy habits into your day-to-day routine, ensuring long-term success without added stress.

CHAPTER 21

Adjusting the Plan for Life's Challenges

How to Handle High-Stress Periods

Even with the best intentions, life inevitably presents high-stress periods that can throw off your cortisol balance and well-being. Whether it's work deadlines, family pressures, or unexpected life events, these challenges can feel overwhelming and have a noticeable impact on your health. However, with the right strategies, you can manage these moments without letting stress take over. The key is to adjust your routine, focus on what you can control, and use practical tools to reduce cortisol spikes and maintain your emotional and physical well-being.

Adjust Your Expectations and Focus on Priorities

In high-stress periods, it's essential to accept that you may not be able to keep up with every element of your routine as planned. Instead of trying to do everything, shift your focus to the essentials that will help you feel balanced and resilient.

- **Identify your non-negotiables**: What are the core habits that keep you grounded? Maybe it's a short meditation session in the morning, a 20-minute walk, or preparing a healthy meal. Focus on maintaining these few key habits that help you manage stress, even if the rest of your routine falls by the wayside.

- **Let go of perfection**: Understand that it's okay if you don't stick to every detail of your plan during high-stress times. Instead, give yourself grace and adjust your expectations. Remember, consistency over time is what matters, not perfection in every moment.

- **Set small, achievable goals**: Break down your routine into smaller tasks that feel manageable. Rather than focusing on completing a full workout, aim for a 10-minute yoga session or a brief walk. These smaller steps still contribute to your overall well-being and help prevent burnout.

Use Quick Stress-Relief Techniques

When you're in the midst of a stressful period, it's important to have quick, effective techniques at your disposal to help calm your nervous system and prevent cortisol levels from spiking.

- **Practice deep breathing exercises**: When you feel stress mounting, take a moment to engage in deep breathing. Slowly inhale for a count of four, hold for four, and exhale for four. This simple technique helps activate your parasympathetic nervous system, reducing stress and cortisol almost immediately.

- **Take short movement breaks**: Even if you can't find time for a full workout, small bursts of movement can help release tension. Stretch, walk around the block, or do a few bodyweight exercises like squats or lunges. Movement helps release endorphins, lowering cortisol levels and improving your mood.

- **Create a calming ritual**: Have a go-to activity that relaxes you, whether it's drinking a cup of herbal tea, listening to calming music, or taking a few minutes for mindfulness. Incorporating a calming ritual, even for just 5-10 minutes, can help reset your stress response.

Fuel Your Body with Cortisol-Friendly Nutrition

High-stress periods often lead to cravings for sugary, processed foods or skipping meals altogether. However, maintaining balanced nutrition is essential for keeping cortisol levels under control.

- **Eat regularly**: Even if you're busy, prioritize regular meals to avoid blood sugar spikes and crashes, which can elevate cortisol. Keep healthy snacks like nuts, seeds, or fruit available to grab when time is tight.

- **Focus on nutrient-dense foods**: Choose meals rich in fiber, lean protein, and healthy fats to support your body during stress. Foods like leafy greens, fatty fish, and avocado provide essential nutrients to regulate cortisol and reduce inflammation.

- **Stay hydrated**: Dehydration can exacerbate stress and increase cortisol levels, so be sure to drink enough water throughout the day. Add lemon or cucumber slices to your water for a refreshing boost.

Prioritize Rest and Sleep

When stress is high, sleep can often be the first thing to suffer, but it's one of the most critical factors in keeping cortisol levels balanced. Prioritize rest as much as possible during high-stress periods.

- **Establish a sleep routine**: Even if your schedule is chaotic, aim to keep a consistent bedtime routine. Turn off screens, dim the lights, and engage in a relaxing pre-sleep ritual like reading or taking a bath.

- **Take restorative breaks**: If you're feeling fatigued during the day, listen to your body and take restorative breaks. Even a 10-minute nap or a brief pause can help recharge your energy and keep cortisol in check.

Ask for Support When Needed

You don't have to handle high-stress periods on your own. Reaching out for help or sharing your challenges with a friend, family member, or coworker can help alleviate some of the emotional load.

- **Communicate your needs**: Let those around you know when you're feeling overwhelmed and need extra support. Whether it's delegating tasks at work or asking for help at home, communicating your needs can ease your stress and prevent cortisol from skyrocketing.

- **Lean on your support system**: Whether it's a friend, partner, or therapist, talking to someone about your stress can be incredibly therapeutic. Sharing your feelings reduces emotional tension, and having someone to listen can make a big difference in how you handle stressful moments.

By incorporating these strategies, you'll be better equipped to handle high-stress periods without letting them derail your cortisol balance or your well-being.

Quick Resets for When Stress Levels Rise Again

Life has a way of throwing unexpected stressors your way, even after you've established a routine for managing cortisol. The good news is that when stress levels spike, you can quickly get back on track with targeted resets that restore balance. These quick resets are designed to be simple and effective, helping you regain control and prevent cortisol from staying elevated for too long.

Use Breathing Techniques to Reset Your Nervous System

One of the fastest ways to lower cortisol in moments of heightened stress is through controlled breathing. Deep breathing activates the parasympathetic nervous system, which naturally lowers stress hormones and helps you feel more grounded.

- **Box breathing**: This method involves inhaling for four seconds, holding your breath for four seconds, exhaling for four seconds, and then holding again for four seconds. Repeat this cycle for 2-3 minutes to quickly calm your body.
- **Alternate nostril breathing**: Another effective technique, this involves closing one nostril and inhaling deeply through the other, then switching sides to exhale. This method balances the nervous system and can bring quick relief during stressful moments.

Take a Mini-Movement Break

When stress spikes, it can create tension in your body. A quick movement break can help release this tension and reset both your physical and mental state.

- **Stretching**: Simple stretches like reaching for the ceiling, touching your toes, or doing gentle spinal twists can instantly reduce muscle tension and improve circulation.
- **Walking**: Even a 5-minute walk outside or around your home can make a big difference. Walking boosts endorphins and helps clear your mind, lowering cortisol and improving mood.

Hydrate and Replenish

Dehydration can increase cortisol levels and exacerbate feelings of stress. When you're in a high-stress period, staying hydrated is essential for keeping cortisol in check.

- **Drink water with electrolytes**: Add a pinch of sea salt or an electrolyte tablet to your water to quickly rehydrate and balance minerals, which can help regulate stress responses.
- **Sip on herbal tea**: Calming teas like chamomile, peppermint, or lemon balm are great for reducing cortisol. Take a few moments to sip on a warm cup of herbal tea and focus on relaxing while hydrating.

Engage in a Quick Mindfulness Reset

Mindfulness helps you anchor yourself in the present moment, making it an effective tool when stress becomes overwhelming. By focusing on the present, you can reduce the mental chatter that contributes to cortisol spikes.

- **5-minute body scan**: Close your eyes and mentally scan your body from head to toe, noticing any areas of tension or discomfort. Focus on relaxing each area as you go. This mindful practice can help release both physical and mental stress.

- **Gratitude practice**: Shift your focus from stress to gratitude by taking a few moments to mentally list three things you're grateful for. Gratitude has been shown to lower cortisol and increase feelings of well-being.

Nourish Yourself with Cortisol-Balancing Snacks

When cortisol levels rise, your body may crave sugary or processed foods, but these can worsen stress. Instead, reach for cortisol-friendly snacks that provide stable energy and support hormone balance.

- **A handful of almonds or walnuts**: These nuts are rich in magnesium, which helps regulate cortisol and promote relaxation.
- **Greek yogurt with berries**: This combination provides probiotics for gut health and antioxidants to combat stress. The protein in yogurt also helps stabilize blood sugar, preventing cortisol spikes.

Disconnect to Reconnect

In today's digital world, constant notifications and information overload can contribute to heightened stress. Taking a brief digital detox can help you reset your mind and lower cortisol levels.

- **Turn off notifications**: Silence your phone or computer notifications for 10-15 minutes. Use this time to disconnect from external demands and focus on yourself.
- **Step away from screens**: Whether it's your phone, computer, or TV, stepping away from screens for even a short time can reduce mental overstimulation and give your brain a break.

Practice Quick Self-Compassion

It's easy to be hard on yourself when stress rises again, but being self-critical only adds to the burden. Instead, practice quick self-compassion to reset your mindset and approach challenges with more resilience.

- **Positive self-talk**: Remind yourself that stress is a natural part of life, and it's okay to have moments where things feel overwhelming. Be kind to yourself and acknowledge that you're doing your best in a challenging situation.
- **Self-compassion pause**: When stress feels intense, take a moment to place your hand over your heart and remind yourself that you deserve care and kindness. This simple gesture can help calm your nervous system and lower cortisol levels.

By using these quick resets during stressful periods, you can prevent prolonged cortisol spikes and regain a sense of control. These techniques are designed to fit into even the busiest days, offering simple but effective tools to support your mental and physical well-being.

Embracing Long-Term Wellness and Sustainable Change

Reflecting on Your 28-Day Journey

As you reach the end of your 28-day journey, it's important to take a moment to reflect on how far you've come. Over the past few weeks, you've committed to not only detoxifying your body from stress-inducing cortisol but also learning strategies to maintain balance and vitality in your everyday life. Whether the changes you experienced were subtle or significant, this journey was about more than just immediate results—it was about laying the foundation for lifelong health.

Celebrating Small Wins

Throughout this process, you likely encountered moments of doubt, fatigue, or even setbacks. But what matters most is your perseverance and your willingness to continue moving forward. Reflect on the small wins you've achieved along the way:

- **Increased energy levels**: Even if every day wasn't perfect, perhaps you noticed moments when you felt more energized and focused, especially after making dietary adjustments and incorporating daily movement.
- **Improved stress management**: Implementing breathing exercises or mindful pauses throughout your day might have helped you feel more in control of your stress response. These tools are not only quick fixes but long-term strategies for keeping cortisol in check.
- **Healthier eating habits**: Whether you followed the meal plans exactly or made modifications that worked for your lifestyle, you likely found that incorporating nutrient-dense, anti-inflammatory foods made a positive impact on how you felt both physically and mentally.

By focusing on these small wins, you'll realize that even incremental progress is worth celebrating. Each positive step forward creates momentum for ongoing success.

Lessons Learned

This 28-day journey was also an opportunity to learn about yourself—your body, your habits, and how you respond to stress. Think about what lessons you've gained from this experience:

- **Understanding your stress triggers**: Perhaps you've become more aware of the specific situations or environments that elevate your cortisol levels, whether it's work pressures, lack of sleep, or skipping meals. Knowing these triggers allows you to take proactive steps to manage them moving forward.

- **Adapting to change**: Throughout this process, you've learned that making small adjustments—whether in your diet, movement, or daily routines—can lead to meaningful results. Flexibility and consistency are key to maintaining balance over time.

- **Building resilience**: Even on difficult days, you've developed resilience by pushing through challenges, whether it was sticking to your movement routine or practicing self-compassion when things didn't go as planned. This resilience will serve you well beyond these 28 days, as life inevitably throws more challenges your way.

Focusing on the Big Picture

While the 28 days are coming to a close, your health journey doesn't end here. These weeks were designed to help you build sustainable habits that can continue to evolve with you. It's not about achieving perfection; rather, it's about consistently making choices that align with your goals of maintaining balanced cortisol levels and overall well-being.

Think about the larger picture:

- **How do you want to feel moving forward?** Whether it's more energized, less stressed, or in better control of your health, your next steps will depend on the vision you have for yourself in the long term.

- **What new habits will you carry with you?** From meal prepping to practicing mindfulness, consider which habits were most impactful for you and how you can integrate them into your life sustainably.

Reflect on the commitment you've made to your health. Your journey wasn't just about following a strict plan—it was about discovering what works best for you and how you can maintain that balance going forward. Every step you took, no matter how small, has contributed to your greater well-being and vitality.

Moving forward, remember to be kind to yourself, celebrate the progress you've made, and continue evolving in ways that honor your body and your health.

Staying Motivated for Lifelong Health

Staying motivated for lifelong health is about much more than short-term goals or temporary fixes—it's about creating a mindset that sustains you for years to come. The habits you've developed over the last 28 days are just the beginning, and keeping your motivation high requires a blend of self-compassion, flexibility, and a focus on what truly matters: feeling your best, long-term. Here's how you can keep that momentum going and ensure your health journey continues to thrive.

Set Meaningful and Realistic Goals

One of the most powerful ways to stay motivated is to set goals that genuinely matter to you. Instead of focusing solely on physical outcomes, like weight loss or muscle tone, think about how you want to feel in your everyday life.

- **Focus on how health impacts your quality of life**: Do you want more energy to play with your kids? Are you aiming to reduce stress so you can focus better at work? When your goals are linked to your deeper desires—like living with vitality, reducing anxiety, or being more present in your relationships—it becomes easier to stay motivated even when challenges arise.

- **Break your goals into manageable steps**: Rather than setting overwhelming, long-term goals, break them into smaller, actionable steps. For example, if your goal is to reduce stress, you could start by scheduling 10 minutes of mindfulness practice into your daily routine. These small steps lead to consistent progress over time.

Build a Routine That Fits Your Life

One of the biggest obstacles to maintaining health habits is feeling like they don't fit into your busy lifestyle. But the key to staying motivated is building a routine that works for you, not against you.

- **Adapt your routine to your lifestyle**: Life can get hectic, and flexibility is crucial. If you can't find time for a 30-minute workout, adjust by doing a 10-minute one instead. If meal prepping for an entire week feels too ambitious, focus on just prepping for the next two days. What matters most is that your routine feels doable and sustainable.

- **Prioritize consistency over perfection**: You're not going to follow your plan perfectly every day—and that's okay. Instead of aiming for perfection, focus on consistency. Missing a workout or indulging in a treat doesn't mean you've fallen off track. What counts is how quickly you return to your healthy habits afterward.

Find Joy in the Process

Health isn't just a destination; it's a journey that should be enjoyable. If your routine feels like a chore, it will be harder to stay motivated. The secret is to find activities that you genuinely enjoy.

- **Choose activities that make you feel good**: Whether it's a brisk walk, yoga, swimming, or dancing, find forms of movement that bring you joy. The more you enjoy your daily health habits, the more likely you'll stick with them long-term.

- **Celebrate small victories**: Motivation thrives when you recognize and celebrate progress. Did you manage to fit in your workouts this week, even if they were shorter than usual? Did you make healthier food choices at a social event? These are all wins worth celebrating, and acknowledging them can boost your motivation to keep going.

Surround Yourself with Support

Accountability and support are essential in maintaining motivation. You don't have to go on this journey alone—surrounding yourself with people who encourage you can make a huge difference.

- **Find an accountability partner**: Whether it's a friend, partner, or family member, having someone to check in with can help keep you on track. Share your goals and celebrate each other's progress.

- **Join a community**: Consider joining a health-focused group or community, whether it's in-person or online. Surrounding yourself with like-minded individuals who are also prioritizing their health can provide extra motivation and inspiration.

Stay Flexible and Kind to Yourself

Life is unpredictable, and your health journey won't always be smooth. There will be times when stress, responsibilities, or unexpected events make it hard to stay on track. During these moments, it's crucial to remain flexible and kind to yourself.

- **Be adaptable**: When life throws you off course, adjust your plan. Instead of feeling guilty for missing a workout or not sticking to a meal plan, ask yourself how you can get back on track in a way that feels manageable. This flexibility allows you to continue making progress without feeling overwhelmed.

- **Practice self-compassion**: On challenging days, remind yourself that health is a long-term journey, not a sprint. Be compassionate with yourself, and acknowledge that setbacks are a normal part of the process. What matters most is your ability to keep moving forward, no matter how small the steps.

By focusing on these strategies, you'll be able to stay motivated for lifelong health, creating a sustainable, enjoyable, and flexible routine that supports your well-being for years to come.

Index of Recipes

Your Exclusive Bonus

Scan the QR-CODE below and get your exclusive bonus!

If you encounter any difficulties accessing the resources,
you can write to us via email at this address: info@heron-books.net

We will be happy to provide you with all the necessary assistance.

Printed in Great Britain
by Amazon

52326691R00084